Library of
Davidson College

FORENSIC PSYCHIATRY

**A Practical Guide for
Lawyers and Psychiatrists**

Publication Number 982

AMERICAN LECTURE SERIES®

A Monograph in

The BANNERSTONE DIVISION *of*
AMERICAN LECTURES IN BEHAVIORAL SCIENCE AND LAW

Edited by

RALPH SLOVENKO, B.E., LL.B., M.A., Ph.D.

Wayne State University
Law School
Detroit, Michigan

FORENSIC PSYCHIATRY

A Practical Guide For
Lawyers And Psychiatrists

By

ROBERT L. SADOFF, M.D.

*Associate Professor of Clinical Psychiatry
Director, Center for Studies in Social-Legal Psychiatry
University of Pennsylvania
Lecturer in Law
Villanova University School of Law
Villanova, Pennsylvania*

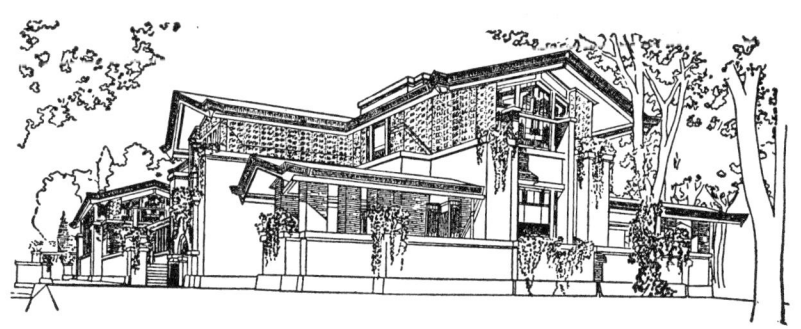

CHARLES C THOMAS • PUBLISHER
Springfield • Illinois • U.S.A.

Published and Distributed Throughout the World by
CHARLES C THOMAS • PUBLISHER
Bannerstone House
301-327 East Lawrence Avenue, Springfield, Illinois, U.S.A.

This book is protected by copyright. No part of it
may be reproduced in any manner without written
permission from the publisher.

© 1975, by CHARLES C THOMAS • PUBLISHER
ISBN 0-398-03412-5
Library of Congress Catalog Card Number: 74-34334

With THOMAS BOOKS careful attention is given to all details of manufacturing and design. It is the Publisher's desire to present books that are satisfactory as to their physical qualities and artistic possibilities and appropriate for their particular use. THOMAS BOOKS will be true to those laws of quality that assure a good name and good will.

Printed in the United States of America
C-1

Library of Congress Cataloging in Publication Data

Sadoff, Robert L.
   Forensic psychiatry.

   (American lecture series, publication no. 982)
   Includes bibliographical references and index.
  1. Forensic psychiatry. I. Title. [DNLM: 1. Forensic psychiatry. W740 S126f]
KF8965.S2   614'.19   74-34334
ISBN 0-398-03412-5

To Joan

FOREWORD

Is PSYCHIATRY too good for the law? Is law too good for psychiatry? Do they simply not go together, like some chemicals? We need not be reminded that many psychiatrists are dissatisfied with the legal process, and many lawyers are dissatisfied with psychiatrists as expert witnesses.

David L. Bazelon, Judge on the United States Court of Appeals for the District of Columbia Circuit for the past twenty-five years, calls psychiatry "the ultimate wizardry." He recently said,

> My experience has shown that in no case is it more difficult to elicit productive and reliable expert testimony than in cases that call on the knowledge and practice of psychiatry. . . . The discipline of psychiatry has direct relevance to cases involving human behavior. One might hope that psychiatrists would open up their reservoirs of knowledge in the courtroom. Unfortunately in my experience they try to limit their testimony to conclusory statements couched in psychiatric terminology. Thereafter they take shelter in a defensive resistance to questions about the facts that are or ought to be in their possession. They thus refuse to submit their opinions to the scrutiny that the adversary process demands.[*]

In an earlier time, two decades ago, Judge Bazelon was not so critical of psychiatrists. He probably feels that he was led down a primrose path by the psychiatric community. Innumerable psychiatrists had declared that, if the law would let them, they could give a more adequate account of realities. They complained, among other things, that the *M'Naghten* test of criminal responsibility restricted their testimony. Judge Bazelon listened, and he responded. To provide juries with "wider horizons

---

[*] D. L. Bazelon, "Psychiatrists and the Adversary Process," *Scientific American* (June 1974), p. 18.

of knowledge concerning mental life," he formulated in the *Durham* case, in 1954, with the aid of psychiatrists, a new test of criminal responsibility. "Its purpose," Judge Bazelon said, "was to bring into the courtroom the knowledge psychiatrists do have." It would, he said, "unfreeze what knowledge psychiatrists do have, to irrigate a field parched by lack of information."

The response of many psychiatrists to the new rule was enthusiastic. Dr. Karl Menninger, one of the patriarchs, described the decision as "more revolutionary" than the *Brown* decision, also rendered in 1954, that outlawed racial segregation in public schools. The enthusiasm though was short-lived. In operation the *Durham* rule turned out to be a fiasco. Dr. Menninger called for psychiatrists to stay out of the courtroom entirely. Judge Bazelon, in speeches and articles, went on a rampage against psychiatrists, much to the annoyance of many psychiatrists.

But what was really to be expected? To call for a psychiatric history in the courtroom replicates a cartoon showing an elderly husband and wife at dinner, the husband saying, "This being our fifty-fifth anniversary, would you like me to summarize?" The late Dr. Winfred Overholser once advised Judge Bazelon that it would take fifty to one hundred hours to furnish the information he wanted. Assuming there is the time for even a summary, what information would be included? What would be relevant? The accused's relationship to his mother? His masturbatory fantasies when he was a boy? If Judge Bazelon had obtained this information, in a fifty or one hundred-hour diagnostic report, he probably would have been more disappointed with it than with the conclusory labels that he got. A diagnostic effort has to be in relation to the disposition. There is a saying, "Don't bite off more than you can chew."

Indeed, the court, as a legal institution, is really not interested in "the truth, the whole truth, and nothing but the truth." It is not curious about much of what the witness could tell. The life of the judicial process is composed of artifacts. They are facts skewed by a script. But to say that the parameters of the law mark out an artificial world is not to debunk the judicial process.

Jack B. Weinstein, Professor of Law at Columbia University and now United States District Court Judge, states:[2]

> The trier's as well as an artist's success in recreating a world must be tested within the frame of reference being used. The law is not interested in the "whole truth" but only in the evidence on the propositions of fact it seems material. This simplification of the issues is, in most instances, a great convenience to the trier, enormously reducing his burdens since so many possible factual issues are immaterial and so much evidence is irrelevant.
>
> Nevertheless, the lack of congruence between the artificial world of the law and that seen by laymen or experts sometimes creates severe problems at a trial. For example, a great part of the debate between doctors and lawyers about the legal definition of insanity and its use by doctors has its source in this incongruity. The frame of reference for the doctor is diagnosis for purpose of treatment while that of the law is judgment for the purpose, among others, of deterrence. Similarly, the lawyer or judge often must struggle with the witness to get to the "facts in the case," by which is meant what the law thinks important, not what the witness cares about.
>
> When fact-finding problems result from the creation of an artificial world which is too far removed from reality, one remedy is to reform the substantive law. For example, the concepts of "fault" or "cause" in automobile collision cases and "insanity" in criminal cases result in problems of proof which might be avoided by rules providing for universal compensation or treatment instead of punishment in civil and criminal cases, respectively. Where the clash is not resolved substantively, the courts attempt to deal with it by relaxing perfectly logical rules of admissibility, thereby permitting the trier to bridge the gap by forcing the law, the facts, or both. Such problems can hardly be solved by general rules of evidence.

To master the script or frame of reference being used in the courts is the function of much of the writing in forensic psychiatry. Most books on forensic psychiatry attempt to show how psychiatry and the law are alike and how they are different; many of these books are used as textbooks for courses in forensic psychiatry in medical and law schools.

This book by Dr. Robert L. Sadoff is written especially for the practicing attorney and for psychiatrists who need to know

---

2. J. B. Weinstein, "Some Difficulties in Devising Rules for Determining Truth in Judicial Trials," *Colum. L. Rev.*, 66:223, 1966.

how to work with each other. It offers a practical approach based on the author's experiences in consulting with lawyers in a variety of cases, both civil and criminal. It is primarily a guide for lawyers about psychiatry, about psychiatrists and how they work, and how psychiatrists may function within the legal system. At the same time it is useful for the practicing psychiatrist who more likely than not will be called for consultation in legal matters at some time in his professional career.

The book covers a number of complex areas of the law in which mental disorder is involved. In the criminal law these include criminal responsibility, competency to stand trial, predictions of dangerousness, and dispositional recommendations for those adjudged delinquent or criminal. In the civil law these include competency, commitment procedures, psychic trauma, workmen's compensation, domestic relations matters, alcohol and drug abuse.

The book is not highly esoteric, but quite pragmatic. With clarity and detail, Dr. Sadoff introduces the attorney to the functions of a psychiatrist in his arena, as well as within the judicial system. Cases are cited for the use of the lawyer. And case examples are presented as an aid to the psychiatrist. By this practical approach, Dr. Sadoff hopes to encourage young psychiatrists to shed their fears of the law and to work more intensively in forensic psychiatry. And by this approach, Dr. Sadoff hopes to aid attorneys in understanding psychiatric examinations and evaluations, and to encourage consultation with psychiatrists in appropriate cases, so the client may obtain a most helpful legal service.

Dr. Sadoff is one of the leaders in the growing field of law and psychiatry. His energy, his enthusiasm, his ebullience, his encouragement of others, his emphasis on the positive, make him a cherished colleague. He is Past President of the American Academy of Psychiatry and Law. He is Associate Professor of Clinical Psychiatry and Director of the Center for Studies in Social-Legal Psychiatry at the University of Pennsylvania, and Lecturer in Law at the Villanova University School of Law. He has written extensively on forensic psychiatry.

RALPH SLOVENKO

ACKNOWLEDGMENTS

THIS BOOK IS A PRODUCT of the experience and training that I have had in forensic psychiatry over the past decade. I am greatly indebted to my teachers, who both trained and stimulated me in this complex and often difficult field. To Melvin S. Heller, M.D. and Samuel Polsky, LL.B., Ph.D., Co-directors of the Unit in Law and Psychiatry at Temple University, I am most indebted for the opportunity of working with them, learning with and from them, and sharing many of the experiences presented in this volume. I am most grateful to the editor, Professor Ralph Slovenko, who has encouraged me in this work and whose careful eye has contributed to its final form. Also to Dennis Koson, M.D., forensic psychiatrist, former student and Fellow, I am deeply grateful for the time he spent reviewing and modifying the manuscript. I wish to thank the publishers of the various journals that originally published some of the chapters in this book and who graciously gave permission to adapt them for publication here.

To my wife and family I am grateful for the time they were deprived of in order for me to complete this book. And to my secretary, Pat Slavick, who began typing some of these chapters as long as five and six years ago, and who has stayed with the project with devotion and stimulation, hours of rereading and retyping, I am especially grateful.

The National Institute of Mental Health has funded our training program in legal psychiatry at the University of Pennsylvania for two and one-half years, under Training Grant Number 2-T21-MH-12883-02. I am most grateful for their cooperation and assistance.

R.L.S.

CONTENTS

Foreword vii
Acknowledgments xi

SECTION I: THE PSYCHIATRIST AND THE LAW

Chapter 1: PSYCHIATRY AND THE LAWYER 5
Chapter 2: THE PSYCHIATRIST AS CONSULTANT IN CIVIL AND CRIMINAL MATTERS 18
Chapter 3: THE PSYCHIATRIC INTERVIEW IN FORENSIC EVALUATIONS 25
Chapter 4: PSYCHIATRIC CONSULTATION WITH REFERRING ATTORNEY IN PREPARATION FOR TRIAL 32
Chapter 5: THE PSYCHIATRIST IN THE COURTROOM 47
Chapter 6: PSYCHIATRIC INVOLVEMENT IN THE SEARCH FOR TRUTH 59

SECTION II: THE PSYCHIATRIST AND CRIMINAL LAW

Chapter 7: MENTAL ILLNESS AND THE CRIMINAL PROCESS: ROLE OF THE PSYCHIATRIST 73
Chapter 8: CRIMINAL BEHAVIOR MASKING MENTAL ILLNESS . 86
Chapter 9: THE PSYCHIATRIST AND DANGEROUSNESS: PREDICTING VIOLENT BEHAVIOR 95
Chapter 10: THE PSYCHIATRIST AND THE JUVENILE IN CRIMINAL PROCEEDINGS 109
Chapter 11: CLINICAL OBSERVATIONS ON PARRICIDE 116
Chapter 12: SEXUALLY DEVIATED OFFENDERS 127
Chapter 13: ALCOHOL AND DRUGS 141

SECTION III: THE PSYCHIATRIST AND CIVIL LAW

Chapter 14: PSYCHIATRIC ASSESSMENT OF MENTAL COMPETENCY 151
Chapter 15: PSYCHIATRIC CONSULTATION IN DOMESTIC RELATIONS MATTERS 159
Chapter 16: A PSYCHIATRIC VIEW OF INSANITY IN ANNULMENT AND DIVORCE 169
Chapter 17: COMMITMENT PROCEDURES 177
Chapter 18: THE PSYCHIATRIST AND THE EVALUATION OF TRAUMA 184

SECTION IV: THE LAW AND THE PSYCHIATRIST

Chapter 19: LEGAL RESPONSIBILITIES OF THE PSYCHIATRIST . . 205
Chapter 20: CONFIDENTIALITY AND PRIVILEGE 211

Glossary 225
Index 247

FORENSIC PSYCHIATRY

A Practical Guide for Lawyers and Psychiatrists

SECTION I

THE PSYCHIATRIST AND THE LAW

THIS SECTION COVERS a number of practical applications of psychiatric consultation in legal matters. Concepts of psychiatry are presented and how psychiatrists function both within psychiatry and in the legal system. I have attempted to spell out, both for attorneys and for psychiatrists working in the law, exactly what procedures and methods are recommended in various tasks the psychiatrist is asked to perform within the judicial system. I am especially concerned with the relationship between the psychiatrist and the lawyer working together to effect a proper and just decision for the client. I have attempted to take the psychiatrist and lawyer together through the various stages of their mutual endeavours in order to effect an optimal functioning of both within a very complex system. Most attorneys have had very little experience working with psychiatrists and most psychiatrists are frightened of legal matters in which they may become involved. Hopefully these chapters will aid the more effective functioning of both attorneys and psychiatrists in working together.

Chapter 1

PSYCHIATRY AND THE LAWYER

PSYCHIATRY IS THAT BRANCH of medicine dealing with mental illness, emotional problems and personality disorders. The psychiatrist is a physician trained to evaluate and treat these conditions. Most psychiatrists view mental illness in the medical model as an illness. Others see it as a social deviance, with psychiatrists serving as social engineers rather than as physicians caring for mentally ill people.

Psychiatrists are trained to detect aberrant personality functioning or deviant behavior in individuals and label them as having psychosis, psychoneurosis or personality disorder. Other forms of diagnoses include the psychophysiological reactions, organic brain disorders and mental retardation.

Psychosis is usually defined as a major mental illness in which the individual experiences a break with reality. Often he is dealing in his own fantasy world or internalized set of beliefs, rather than those shared by society or his immediate community. The major psychoses are schizophrenia and the affective psychoses, including depression and manic-depressive illness.

The psychoneuroses are also considered to be forms of mental illness of a less severe nature than the psychoses, but may be equally as crippling or incapacitating. All psychoneuroses have a common element of anxiety at their core. The major ones include:

anxiety neurosis
phobic neurosis
obsessive-compulsive neurosis
depressive neurosis
depersonalization neurosis
hypochondriacal neurosis

hysterical neurosis of which there are two types:
  conversion
  dissociative.

Personality disorders are described in the Diagnostic and Statistical Manual II (DSM II).[1] These disorders are aberrant types of personality configurations which are not normal and often are associated with personal or social difficulties. The personality disorders are listed as follows:

  paranoid personality
  cyclothymic personality
  schizoid personality
  explosive personality
  obsessive-compulsive personality
  hysterical personality
  asthenic personality
  antisocial personality
  passive-aggressive personality
  inadequate personality.

These personality disorders are found in individuals who have difficulties at work, with other people, and often come to the attention of psychiatrists because of legal involvement. Most people have a personality type which can be described but is not necessarily a disorder. There are personality traits as well as personality disorders.

It might be well at this point to define briefly general conceptualizations in psychiatry.

  A. Mind-body dichotomy

   The mind is a nonphysical conceptualization of thought processes, behavior and responses to stimuli. The brain is composed of nerve cells and other tissues. The mind is separate from the body but also related to it. The mind can influence body functions and can be influenced by physical actions and behavior. A disturbed mind may lead to disorders of the body, such as ulcers, high blood pressure, ulcerative colitis, etc. This is mediated through the mechanism of anxiety; anxiety is not "fear," but a person who has fear may show anxiety. Similarly, if the body is hurt, traumatized or stressed, the mind will be affected. Confusion, poor judgment, memory loss or irritability may be noted.

B. Personality

Personality is a conceptualization in psychiatry which refers to the totality of attitudes and behaviors of an individual based on his experiences from early infancy. There are certain types of personalities described according to principal features. Some types of personalities are

    obsessive-compulsive   histrionic
    aggressive   introverted
    passive   extroverted

These personalities may be "normal" in the sense that they are not personality disorders. These personality traits do not usually result in anxiety and the individual is able to function fairly effectively. He will be characterized, however, by a personality type which differentiates him from others. The analogy is similar in music; there are certain basic notes that are played but the overtimes characterize the specific features of a tone. People are basically similar, but the overtones of their personalities identify their individuality.*

C. Stress

Stress upon individuals will vary with different types of personality configurations. Stress to any part of a person's body will result in a reaction to his psyche. The basic mechanism of this reaction is *regression*. The person who in injured will regress; the person who is under emotional tension and in need of support will also show regression; i.e. a backward movement to an earlier stage of his psychological development. Thus, a person who functions at a fairly mature level may regress to an earlier stage and appear at times during the period of stress to be immature,

---

* A fuller description of all diagnostic labels may be found in DSM-II[1] or Noyes' *Modern Clinical Psychiatry*.[2]

silly or infantile in his mannerisms and behavior. He may show good judgment in decision making that he has shown previously, but he may have seriously regressed reactions to other areas of his life such as his sexual or interpersonal relationships.

There are a number of other *mechanisms of defense* besides regression that an individual utilizes while under pressure, stress or trauma. Some of these are (1) *repression:* a person may push the trauma down into the unconscious, thereby forgetting or showing "amnesia" for an event. (2) *Compensation:* an individual may overcompensate for his feelings of inadequacy by being or appearing "supernormal." (3) *Conversion* is a common form of defense mechanism or adaptation to stress that people with hysterical personality configurations may utilize, and one may see conversion reactions in which an individual experiences or expresses physical disability when no organic cause exists. This is due to the conversion of the psychic conflict into a physical symptom so often noted in accident or negligence cases.

This is a brief description of elementary psychological principles the attorney may encounter in his work with mentally ill clients. The section is short and is designed not to burden the practicing lawyer with complex concepts that are difficult to comprehend. For a more detailed description of psychiatric and psychoanalytic concepts, the reader is referred to Watson's *Psychiatry for Lawyers.*[3]

THE PSYCHIATRIST AND THE LAWYER

In addition to knowing principles of psychiatry, the attorney ought to understand the variations in psychiatric training leading to various emphases in psychiatry. This understanding may make a substantial difference in the attorney's choice of a psychiatrist for a particular medical-legal evaluation.

Perhaps the most widely publicized form of psychiatric training is the psychoanalytically oriented type which follows the teachings of Sigmund Freud. The Freudian psychiatrist is one who views people in a psychodynamic light, attempting to understand individual behavior on the basis of intrapersonal psychodynamic conflicts. He would be more inclined to consider psychic determinism, i.e. that a person does not really have free will, but that his behavior is predicated upon his earlier experiences and childhood conflicts. Thus, he may be inclined, e.g. toward a view of lack of criminal responsibility. (The defendant could not help himself, he was found to do it because of earlier emotional conflicts.) However, this view is compounded by the fact that Freud himself warned against the use of psychoanalytic concepts in courtroom situations. He considered psychoanalysis both a tool for exploring human behavior and for therapy of psychological problems. He did not consider it appropriate for invasion into the courtroom. Most psychoanalysts are not inclined toward forensic work.

A second form of training is that in behavior therapy principles following the Pavlovian conditioning response. Treatment is based upon deconditioning, desensitization to specific stimuli which cause excessive anxiety or phobic symptoms. The behavior therapist is mostly involved in the treatment of specific types of illness and usually does not become involved in legal matters.

The organically oriented psychiatrist, or neuropsychiatrist, has had a significant place in forensic work. Most commonly, the neuropsychiatrist, i.e. the physician who is trained in both neurology and psychiatry, has been called for examination of psychophysiological reactions following trauma, to determine the etiology of specific symptoms which may be functional, organic or malingered. The neuropsychiatrist is most likely to view behavior as being due to organic or biologic causes. He is less likely than the psychoanalyst to consider the psychodynamic conflicts which could prevent or inhibit freedom of will. Many organically oriented psychiatrists treat people with such forms of therapy as chemotherapy (drugs), electroshock therapy or psychosurgery, if needed.

Attorneys ought to be aware that most psychiatrists will attempt to be honest and scientifically neutral in their approach, but their evaluations will depend in great part upon both their experience and their own personal backgrounds. Thus we find a number of psychiatrists who "always" testify for defense or those who "always" testify for the prosecution. On the civil side we have those who are considered to be defendant's psychiatrists and those who are plaintiff's psychiatrists. It is important, in my opinion, for a psychiatrist to be available to either side, to evaluate and possibly testify for defense or plaintiff in civil cases, and similarly for prosecution or defense in criminal cases. To become labeled as a psychiatrist who is almost exclusively a defense psychiatrist is something that will negatively affect the image of that psychiatrist and make his evaluations less credible. The important criterion in a psychiatric examination, because it is so highly subjective, is the credibility of the psychiatrist. That is, how valid, how believeable are his conclusions based on the skills of his interview and assessment of the problems.

A number of psychiatrists may arrive at the same diagnosis medically, the same psychodynamic factors affecting behavior, but the application of the medical findings to legal tests or legal standards causes psychiatrists a bit of difficulty. It is this difficulty in application to legal concepts which often emerges in the press as the major reason for disagreement among psychiatrists. This is not to say that psychiatrists do not disagree upon diagnosis or etiology, or other medical issues, because we do, but the emphasis is often placed on the lack of psychiatric agreement in applying medical findings to legal criteria.

It is important also for the attorney to understand that people change from time to time, from day to day, and that a diagnosis of schizophrenia made legitimately at one point in a person's life may not be made if the outstanding features of that illness do not emerge on subsequent evaluation and only the residual features or personality disorder is apparent.

Thus we have people who have been through hospitalizations and evaluations over a number of years with several diagnoses including schizophrenia, manic-depressive reaction, anxiety reaction, phobic reaction, passive-aggressive personality, schizoid personality and/or inadequate personality. These labels all may be ascribed to the same individual, but the person evaluating that individual is different, his interview is different, the time is different, the patient himself may focus on or emphasize different features in his personality which will lead the psychiatrist to a different diagnosis or a different conclusion.

It is certainly true that two psychiatrists examining the same patient at the same time may come up with different diagnoses. For example, a prominent forensic psychiatrist and the author both examined a defendant in a criminal case in a part of the United States away from either of our homes. We both interviewed together in the same room, listening to the patient's story. At the end of a two-hour interview, we compared our findings and diagnoses. His diagnosis was sociopathic personality disorder with paranoid features. I chose to call the patient schizoid personality with paranoid features and sociopathic traits. The man had killed two women, had been apprehended and was struggling to save his life. There was no question that he had antisocial features; there was no question that he had paranoid tendencies, and the author chose also to see his basic personality configuration as that of a schizoid. This is the way he dealt with people on an interpersonal basis. However, his behavior was antisocial and part of his thinking was paranoid. Therefore, he could have three separate diagnoses; the significant aspect was which to emphasize in the diagnostic classification in reporting our findings to the attorneys or the judge. The focus of the labelling may well have an influence on outcome or disposition.

This is something that attorneys have difficulty understanding because psychiatrists have a great deal of difficulty in expressing a particular case. We seem to understand the diagnostic labelling intuitively and have difficulty sharing our experience and knowledge in a verbal manner with our legal colleagues.

The diagnosis, therefore, may be affected by the background of the one making the diagnosis; i.e. is he behaviorally oriented; is he psychodynamically oriented; is he socially oriented; where could he place his focus, on personality configuration or mental illness diagnosis?

The selection of the proper psychiatrist for each case may be very important. However, do we have sufficient forensic psychiatrists or general psychiatrists who are interested in legal work to be available for consultation to attorneys? It may be that the attorney does not have the luxury of choice for particular cases. In some areas, of course, in the larger cities such as New York, Chicago, Detroit, Boston, Philadelphia, San Francisco and Los Angeles, there are a number of well-trained forensic psychiatrists who are available for such consultation.

Specialty Groups

Recently there was formed the American Academy of Psychiatry and the Law, a group now numbering well over three hundred throughout the country and in various parts of the world. This group began in 1969, under the leadership of Dr. Jonas Rappeport and has grown considerably to the present. Primarily the group is composed of psychiatrists who are interested in learning from each other as well as sharing their experiences with other psychiatrists and attorneys throughout the country.

Another group which includes psychiatrists working in forensic areas is the American Academy of Forensic Sciences, a group with a much broader scope, incorporating not only psychiatrists, but physicians, attorneys and forensic scientists of all types, providing a more comprehensive approach to medical-legal problems. A third group is the American College of Legal Medicine, comprised primarily of dually degreed individuals, physicians and attorneys, who work primarily in the fields of legal medicine, specifically medical malpractice cases and other areas in which physicians and attorneys are likely to encounter each other.

Most of these groups have directories of psychiatrists and members who may be called upon for consultation or advice by attorneys wishing aid in particular problems. Consulting the directory of the American Academy of Psychiatry and the Law, for example, will give the attorney in any part of the country a fairly comprehensive list of psychiatrists who are experienced in legal work.

Training in Legal Psychiatry

Training in legal psychiatry is another matter. Most of the forensic psychiatrists have been trained by preceptorship or on-the-job training with their own initiative. During the past ten years or more, however, the National Institute of Mental Health has sponsored the training of forensic psychiatrists in a number of centers around the country. These have been primarily the University of Southern California, University of California at Los Angeles, Temple University, University of Pennsylvania, University of Maryland, University of Pittsburgh and Boston University. These specific fellowships, however, have ended with the change in philosophy of NIMH from that of training elite forensic psychiatrists to the training of general psychiatrists with forensic information.

Recently we did a survey of the type of training that exists in the medical schools in America and found very little teaching of forensic psychiatry to medical students and only little more to psychiatric residents. Most of the training is concentrated in a few centers in the country where forensic psychiatrists abound and have been previously trained. Much of the training occurs at a general level with a few lectures or demonstrations. Psychiatrists are beginning to realize the value and importance of understanding legal considerations because unquestionably, every psychiatrist at one time or another will find himself professionally in court, either aiding a patient or defending himself.

THE PSYCHIATRIST AND THE LAW

It seems fairly accurate to say that it is virtually impossible for the practicing psychiatrist today to avoid involvement in the legal process. In order for the psychiatrist *qua* physician to set up an office he must first be licensed by law. In addition, he must be aware of his legal obligations to his patients, so that he will not be negligent in his practice or be involved in a malpractice suit. For such considerations he must carry adequate amounts of insurance and be aware of legal standards of practice in his area.

The psychiatrist encounters sick patients, some of whom may need to be committed to hospitals. He must know the laws involving involuntary commitment and his responsibility and obligation both to his patients and to his community.

More specifically, the psychiatrist may be called in by the law as a specialist in order to aid in judicial procedures. In criminal procedures he may be called to examine a defendant to determine his competency to stand trial, or his degree of responsibility at the time the crime was committed. Further, the psychiatrist may need to advise the court with respect to dispositional recommendations in criminal procedures; he may even be asked to predict whether a person may commit future violent acts. The range of psychiatric utilization in criminal procedures has been broadened recently and the psychiatrist has become more involved in treating offenders, advising parole and probation officers, and even consulting with state legislatures in the enactment of criminal statutes.

The scope of psychiatric involvement in civil procedures has also been broadened and includes determination of competency for a number of procedures, a variety of domestic relations problems, negligence suits, including post-traumatic emotional conditions and for commitment procedures.

In addition, recently the forensic psychiatrist has become involved in consultation for therapeutic abortion, evaluation and treatment of individuals using and abusing various narcotics and other drugs. Virtually any evaluation which may be utilized in a judicial proceeding is a forensic psychiatric problem. Also, any patient or ex-patient who becomes involved in legal proceedings may involve the treating psychiatrist in a forensic experience for which he ought to be prepared.

A brief survey of psychiatric attitudes toward participation in legal cases clearly indicated that psychiatrists generally are afraid of the law, want nothing to do with lawyers or courts and often mistrust the intentions of the lawyer who calls them. My own experience reveals that most other psychiatrists are delighted to have such "masochistic" colleagues as forensic psychiatrists with whom to consult and refer their legal cases in order to avoid their own involvement.

There are many who decry the role of the psychiatrist in court and say he does not belong there at all. Others have had frustrating and unrewarding or degrading experiences in testifying as expert witnesses and vow never to become involved again. Many psychiatrists are so afraid of legal involvement they would never agree to testify in any legal procedure if they could avoid it.

They point to the unfairness of the trial and the disadvantages a psychiatrist has under cross-examination by an expert at such interrogation. They claim the psychiatrist is not trained to answer the "tricky" questions posed to him and is not really able to handle the situation comfortably.

Many psychiatrists have said that the law is interested only in facts (not in truth) and in the specific methods that have been developed through the years in arriving at these facts. They criticize lawyers and judges for not caring about the individual or his feelings, or about special circumstances that may be involved. They also argue that most lawyers are excessively rigid in their application of the law.

Any psychiatrist may be called upon to examine an individual involved in either a civil or a criminal legal matter and also be required at some time to testify with respect to his opinions as an expert witness. More commonly, the psychiatrist may be asked to produce his records or to testify in the case of a patient whom he is treating. The psychiatrist may decline the invitation to examine a patient for legal purposes, but if he is treating a patient who becomes involved in legal matters, he may have no choice as to whether or not his testimony will be required.

The psychiatrist may also be involved in legal matters when he is sued for negligence or malpractice, e.g. in cases involving involuntary commitment, electroshock therapy, or suicide.

Thus the psychiatrist may become involved in legal procedures through his patients, his own professional conduct and also his own personal conduct. It is not unknown that psychiatrists have become involved in legal difficulties due to personal domestic relations problems, tort action in automobile accidents or perhaps a criminal matter involving abuse of drugs.

Any patient that a doctor is treating may become involved in a criminal matter resulting in the court subpoenaing the records of the doctor. In this case the doctor may not be called in as an expert witness, but as a fact witness as to whether or not the patient discussed the committing of crimes in his therapeutic sessions. If it were found in the doctor's records that the patient had contemplated committing such crimes, what obligation does the physician have to reveal such information to the authorities?

Does he become an accomplice before the fact? Is he withholding material information if he does not produce his records, or if he produces only a part of the records, or if he declines to answer questions about his patient's verbal productions in order to protect his confidential role with the patient?

The classical example of this latter problem was brought dramatically to the surface recently when a young man went to the top of a tower at the University of Texas and began shooting people, killing many. It was reported that he had mentioned such an urge to the school psychiatrist prior to this behavior. How seriously can such utterances be taken? Should action to prevent such behavior be taken in every case when a homicidal or suicidal urge is verbalized in a therapeutic session?

Most psychiatrists feel a tolerance for minor criminal activities, such as shoplifting, smoking marijuana, consensual adult sexual offenses and other nonviolent acts which are construed as symptoms of mental illness or emotional disturbance. To report such behavior to authorities is to undermine the confidence patients have in psychiatrists and prevent such problems from coming to the surface. (Not to mention the effect their revelation has on all current and future patients' confidence in the privacy of their communications to a psychiatrist.) However, most psychiatrists are also of the opinion that murder, armed robbery and other violent crimes are not to be tolerated nor handled only in therapy. Most would attempt to get their patients to confess to the proper authorities if they were certain of the criminal behavior. In the event the patient refuses, however, the psychiatrist will likely terminate therapy with the patient. Certainly the psychiatrist must be careful not to become overly involved in a patient's fantasies of crime or crimes that he says he may have committed in the past. If the psychiatrist can prevent the homicide or danger either to his patient or to a potential victim, he has as much duty to do so as he has to prevent a suicide in his patient.

Perhaps one of the major frustrations that has been enunciated is that there is no compatibility between the law and psychiatry, for the law is geared toward controlling behavior and psychiatry toward understanding it. My own feeling is that where law and psychiatry come together, the issue is not exclusively in controlling or understanding the behavior, but rather in modifying it. The author has found the law will accept the modification of aberrant behavior leading to control of antisocial acts, and psychiatry certainly will go beyond the stage of mere understanding of the behavior and consider modification to prevent further aberrant behavior.

We have seen many misunderstandings between lawyers and psychiatrists with respect to each other's role in court. This book is designed to help clarify these misunderstandings and provide the attorney with a clearer understanding of psychiatry and psychiatrists functioning within the legal system. Many of the problems raised and discussed are based on numerous questions and problems that have been presented to the author by other psychiatrists who are plagued with misunderstanding of their role and expectations in the variety of legal procedures that confront them, and by practicing attorneys who have limited experience in working with psychiatrists.

The purpose of this chapter is to provide a brief introduction to some concepts in psychiatry, the labels we use and the methods by which we approach problems. It is not intended to serve as a substitute for good psychiatric evaluation and it is not intended to make the lawyer into a psychiatrist. (Neither should the psychiatrist attempt to be the attorney.) However, it is felt that the more familiar the attorney is with the ways in which psychiatrists approach problems, the better we will understand each other and the more effective will be the psychiatric consultation within specific legal situations.

REFERENCES

1. *Diagnostic and Statistical Manual of Mental Disorders,* 2d ed. (DSM-II), Washington, D.C., Amer Psychiat Assoc, 1968.
2. Kolb, L. C.: *Noyes' Modern Clinical Psychiatry,* 7th ed. Philadelphia, Saunders, 1968.
3. Watson, A. S.: *Psychiatry for Lawyers.* New York, Intl Univs Press, 1968.

Chapter 2

THE PSYCHIATRIST AS CONSULTANT IN CIVIL AND CRIMINAL MATTERS

IN PREVIOUS ARTICLES the author has described the role of the psychiatrist in criminal[1] and civil[2] procedures and suggested areas of expansion of this role. In this chapter the specific functions of the psychiatrist as consultant in legal matters will be delineated.

1. Psychiatric examination of client/defendant.
2. Evaluation of client/defendant within the legal situation.
3. Collection of information and data necessary and relevant to the legal matter.
4. Collation of this data and integration with examination and evaluation of client/defendant.
5. Interpretation of findings and evaluation.
6. Transmitting this interpretation to attorneys and judges.
7. Presenting this interpretation clearly, properly and relevantly in a courtroom procedure when indicated.

These seven steps are viewed as distinct and discrete and each with its own structure, series of problems and conclusions. Most lawyers would acknowledge the expertise of the psychiatrist to conduct a proper psychiatric examination of the client or defendant. Most attorneys would expect the psychiatrist to be able to evaluate the findings of the examination within the specific legal situation and to be able to transmit these findings to attorneys and to testify to them in court, if called upon. The two steps which are most often overlooked, or neglected, in forensic psychiatric consultations are the investigative, or information

---

This chapter is adapted from an article originally published in the *Pennsylvania Bar Association Quarterly*, entitled "The Psychiatrist as Consultant in Civil and Criminal Law," Vol. XLIII (January, 1972), No. 2, p. 176.

gathering phase and the application of the data collected to the evaluation of the client and interpretation for legal purposes.

The author has found that psychiatrists who have attended law school seem to be more concerned about the investigative phase and need to know as much as possible about the defendant or client and about the legal situation in which he is involved. Generally, however, psychiatrists without legal training or experience are content with the traditional psychiatric examination through interview. The author contends that in criminal cases this is not sufficient, except perhaps when examining for competency to stand trial; i.e. present state of mind.

For determination of criminal responsibility, i.e. mental state at some prior time, it is imperative to have other information in most cases. This information might include interviews with parents, spouse, children, employers, friends or other significant individuals who had observed the defendant at or around the time of the crime. It most often also includes interviewing the arresting officer and receiving a copy of any statement the defendant may have made to police. For example, if the defendant had taken a lie detector test and what were the results. It is important to know about previous hospitalizations or medical examinations prior to or subsequent to the time of the crime. In most cases a complete physical examination and occasionally a neurological examination conducted on the client would be helpful. Very often a comprehensive battery of psychological testing to corroborate findings, to supplement them, or to provide information which is unobtainable clinically, such as minimal evidence for brain damage, or underlying psychotic processes, is necessary. Quite frequently in the event of amnesia,* a sodium amytal® interview should be conducted to ascertain the nature of the amnesia and whether or not further information can be gathered which is not available clinically without the use of amytal.[3]

Many of the author's medical colleagues criticize the need for all of this "extraneous" information. They indicate that a psy-

---

* For a further discussion of amnesia, see Chapter 3. For a more comprehensive presentation and discussion of the use of sodium amytal® and other means of obtaining information, see Chapter 6, "Psychiatric Involvement in the Search for Truth."

chiatrist is not expected to be a lawyer and should confine his examination to the traditional interview technique. Some feel that if the psychiatrist knows too much he becomes biased and cannot render a neutral opinion. Most psychiatrists don't even want to become involved in examining an individual for criminal responsibility. They feel the psychiatrist is in no position to make such a determination, since in many cases the legal criteria for insanity or criminal responsibility involves philosophical doctrines of right and wrong for which the psychiatrist has no expertise. They also indicate that the psychiatrist ought not become involved in criminal matters until after the findings and only then should he testify with respect to dispositional recommendations.

The author feels that the psychiatrist can offer an opinion about criminal responsibility if he has conducted a comprehensive investigation into the matter and not merely an examination of the defendant. Yet, it is true that in some cases the best opinion rendered is that no opinion can be formed about responsibility at the time of the crime, either because necessary information could not be obtained or because of limited expertise and lack of available tools to make an accurate determination.

Two brief examples will highlight the difficulties a limited psychiatric examination may have on the court.

> In one case the author testified that the defendant had been under the belief that his testicles had been removed at age thirteen because he had suffered from the mumps, which involved his testes. Inasmuch as the offense was a sexual one, this information appeared to be significant in the evaluation of the defendant's personality. When the judge wisely asked whether or not the defendant indeed had had such an operation, or had his testicles removed, it was necessary to confess that a thorough physical examination had not been conducted since it was not "a part of the routine psychiatric examination." The court was thereupon recessed for ten minutes so that the defendant could be examined more thoroughly. The results were related to the court whether or not this was indeed

the case or whether the defendant was under a misapprehension.

The second example also occurred in the middle of a trial under cross-examination. Having testified about what the defendant had told the author and what information was gathered, the district attorney asked whether or not the arresting officer had been questioned about his impressions of the defendant at the time of the arrest. Since this had not been done, the judge granted a recess and ordered a meeting with the officer, who was present in the courtroom, to discuss his evaluation of the defendant at the time of arrest (many months prior to this examination of him).

These may seem like insignificant pieces of information in the general evaluation of a defendant, but apparently in both instances they were important to the judge. His expectation was that these examinations had been included in the comprehensive work-up of the defendant.

Too often the psychiatrist, either wanting to please, wishing to show his erudition and his ability to fit complex psychodynamic or theoretical considerations into a practical legal matter, will render an opinion for or against insanity, where the best opinion may have been that within reasonable medical certainty one cannot tell one way or the other.

In many cases there are bona fide differences of opinion with respect to insanity. It has been suggested that the psychiatrists testifying for both sides discuss their opinions among themselves and file an addition to their own opinion; i.e. a joint opinion, concerning the areas where they agree and disagree.

In criminal matters, when the psychiatrist presents recommendations for disposition he should know something about the institutions which are involved in his recommendation; i.e. the psychiatrist must investigate the correctional institutions and find out what type of therapy or rehabilitative measures are available for the inmates and also find out what type of supervision a man might receive on probation or parole, and whether or not he would be able to obtain psychiatric treatment in various institutions while on probation. It is senseless for a psychiatrist to recommend to the court that which is impossible to obtain within the community.

A recent study we conducted on probationed sex offenders finds psychiatric opinion following a series of evaluation and treatment sessions to have greater validity and reliability than that opinion arising out of a single interview.[4] Thus, in criminal matters, the psychiatrist consulting with the law and with the courts on issues of criminal responsibility and in recommendations for disposition, must be well prepared with as much information about the defendant, the legal situation and about the community resources as he can be. To do less is to be an ineffective consultant.

In civil cases, especially in matters of child custody and visitation, and in post-traumatic illness, the consulting psychiatrist must have a comprehensive view of the situation or his opinion is bound to be biased. Unfortunately, in most cases of child custody the psychiatrist is called in by one or the other lawyer, and is not appointed by the court. When this occurs, invariably the other party does not submit to psychiatric examination and only a partial view is obtained. The author feels that it is necessary for the psychiatrist in these matters to have the opportunity of examining the child alone, each parent alone, the parents together and the child in the company of each parent. This multiple examination and evaluation is essential in arriving at an opinion about the child's best interests and welfare as he relates to each of the parents and as they relate to him. This area will be further developed in Chapter 16.

It is essential in domestic relations cases, wherever possible, that all parties involved be examined both alone and in concert, since often the individual factors are not the determining ones but rather the dynamic interrelationship between members of the disrupted family.[5]

In evaluation of a plaintiff in tort action, especially post-traumatic neurosis or psychosis, it behooves the psychiatrist to have as much information as is available on the plaintiff's mental state. The important factor here is the state of mind of the plaintiff prior to the accident, at the time of the accident and subsequent to the trauma. The psychiatrist has to be able to determine whether or not there was preexisting mental illness which either was activated, reactivated, aggravated by the accident; or whether the patient was free of all illness prior to accident and any illness appearing subsequent to the accident was caused by it and not by some stress or other factors unrelated to the accident. The case examples are presented in Chapter 20.

Often we are blinded by the goal which we seek and would be willing to use what is often called "tunnel vision" in order to support our hypothesis. That is, if one needs to conclude that the accident did cause the mental illness, one must be open-minded about looking for alternative causes which are more reasonable and more likely than the accident itself. The narrow view naturally leads to difficulty on cross-examination and inhibits a more comprehensive view of the matter.

Too often the author has been disappointed by attorneys who have withheld information which they felt would have been harmful to their client and expected conclusions favoring their case. What they failed to see is that this information is available and will be used effectively to attack my testimony on cross-examination.

The thrust of this chapter has been to highlight the need for the psychiatrist consulting in legal matters to be provided with as much data or information that he can use to integrate into his examination and evaluation. The other five steps outlined above shall not be dwelled upon. However, concerning the psychiatrist's testimony in court, the author believes in the value of the adversary system and that the consulting psychiatrist should provide as much help as possible to the attorney who consults him. The psychiatrist is the agent of the attorney who calls upon him and will help as much with the examination, evaluation and interpretative stages, as well as provide the attorney with necessary information that can be used in cross-examining witnesses. The psychiatrist's bias should be with the attorney's side in all phases of consultation until he becomes an expert witness. At this point, the psychiatrist ceases to be an agent of the patient/defendant/client, but becomes an agent of the court.

The testimony should be presented in a clear and professional manner as to evince a feeling of credibility from the jury and the judge. One must expect that the testimony will be effectively attacked by competent cross-examination and that any damage done to the testimony will be repaired by proper re-direct examination. In this way the psychiatrist as expert witness does not need to become defensive or argumentative in the courtroom, but can be more properly effective as an educator by sharing with the court the benefit of his experience in psychiatry, and specifically his examination of the client, and comprehensive professional interpretation in the instant case.

The various phases of psychiatric consultation in legal matters have been outlined primarily for the education of the lawyers utilizing psychiatric aid, but also to emphasize the complexity of this role which is not to be taken lightly. Training centers have been established in various parts of the country to provide education, experience and supervision for psychiatrists wishing to become consultants to the law. The role has become so important and complex that only a well-trained and experienced forensic psychiatrist can properly fulfill these complex consultative functions.

REFERENCES

1. Sadoff, R. L.: Mental illness and the criminal process: The role of the psychiatrist. *Am Bar Assoc J, 54*:566, June, 1968.
2. Sadoff, R. L.: Civil law and psychiatry: New dimensions. *Am Bar Assoc J, 56*:165, Feb., 1970.
3. Sadoff, R. L.: Psychiatric involvement in the search for truth. *Am Bar Assoc J, 52*:251, March, 1966.
4. Sadoff, R. L., Roether, H. A., and Peters, J. J.: Clinical measure of enforced group psychotherapy. *Am J Psychiatr, 128*:224, Aug., 1971.
5. Sadoff, R. L.: The expanding role of psychiatric consultation in civil-legal procedures. In Wecht, Cyril (Ed.): *Legal Medicine Annual.* New York, Appleton, 1970.

Chapter 3

THE PSYCHIATRIC INTERVIEW IN FORENSIC EVALUATIONS

THIS CHAPTER WILL OUTLINE in detail the psychiatric approach to the defendant who is examined in a criminal proceeding.

The psychiatric interview should be conducted in a quiet room conducive to concentration and free association. The patient should not fear the room is "bugged" so that others might be listening or watching during the interview. Ideally, he should be interviewed by the psychiatrist alone, but occasionally this is not possible and the defendant's attorney may be present during the examination. Usually this presents no problem for the examiner, unless the attorney attempts to answer questions posed to the patient.

By all means the psychiatrist ought to identify himself to the patient and explain to him exactly what is his role. Too often this is not done and the patient does not know whom the psychiatrist may represent. If the psychiatrist is called in by defense counsel, he should so state and indicate what are the purposes of the examination. Similarly, if the psychiatrist is called in by the government (or prosecution) or by the court as a neutral examiner, he should identify his position and role to the defendant/client/patient. The well-trained forensic psychiatrist usually has no difficulty in communicating with defendants from lower socioeconomic backgrounds. His experience and training in forensic psychiatry has exposed him to a great number of individuals from various backgrounds.

Initially, the psychiatrist attempts to put the patient at ease by a few atraumatic questions and comments about neutral situations and gradually builds up to the more critical issues involved. With respect to forensic psychiatric examinations in criminal cases, however, it has been found helpful to proceed almost directly to the reasons for the individual being confined or examined at that time. For example, the psychiatrist may ask the patient, "Do you know why you are being examined by a psychiatrist?" Or, "How long have you been in prison?" Or, "Why have you been confined to this prison?" This type of questioning usually leads into the critical material necessary for examination of current mental status as well as an indication of previous mental state at the time of the alleged offense. If so, a full discussion of the instant offense is pursued—the patient's recollection of it, his version of it as compared with the official version which the psychiatrist has reviewed prior to the interview. This matter is dealt with in great detail by having the patient narrate the situation to the examiner with a few questions interspersed.

The next important component of the interview is a questioning in detail of past medical history, past personal and social history in order to determine patterns of behavior, previous medical conditions which are pertinent to the current state of mind, and family history which reflects attitudes as well as facts about siblings, parents and medical complications. Previous mental difficulties or emotional traumata in childhood, with dream material, where obtainable, is requested by the interviewer. The patient's attitudes, concerns and feelings are examined along with the content of the interview. This is an important consideration to keep in mind. The examination is not merely what the patient says, but how he presents the material with attendant feelings, attitudes, mood, behavior and spontaneous physical or verbal responses.

Following a lengthy discussion of his past history and his current personal attitude, a return to the instant offense is developed with strict questioning by the examiner to obtain clarity, to search for inconsistencies and to develop patterns.

The review of mental status aspects is an essential feature of the first interview with an evaluation of the patient's appearance, including dress, attitude, posture, approach to questions, his behavior (e.g. does he smoke?) and how he responds to various critical questions.

Next is an evaluation of his intellectual capacities, affective responses, his mood, his orientation; i.e. does he know where he is, who he is and the time, does he show mental confusion, is he aware of the nature of the situation in which he is involved? Specific questions regarding the instant offense also will indicate whether he has present mental capacity; i.e. mental competency to stand trial. Does he know the nature of the charges in which he is involved, the consequences thereof and what could befall him if he were found guilty of the charges? Is he able to communicate effectively during the interview such that it is likely he could communicate effectively with counsel in preparing a rational defense? Also, does he possess sufficient strength to be able to withstand the rigors of trial such that he would not deteriorate to a psychotic condition at time of trial?

The first interview will reveal to the examiner the state of mind of the individual at the time he is examined, with some indications as to his state of mind at the previous time for which he is alleged to have committed a crime. It will also give the examiner the defendant's attitude about the crime, about the situation in which he is involved, review of past personal, familial, social, vocational, educational and medical histories, along with a tentative diagnosis or impression with suggestions for treating any illness noted.

All necessary information about the patient and his alleged offense should be reviewed by the psychiatrist prior to his second interview with the patient. If psychological testing is necessary, or if further tests such as electroencephalogram, blood sugar (or other blood chemistry) or skull X rays are necessary, they should be obtained prior to further clinical interviews. By obtaining statements of confession read to the police, by examining others who may have seen the defendant at the time of the alleged offense, or near that time, by discussing the problem with mother, spouse or other close family member, the psychiatrist will have the ability to corroborate certain information received from the patient or to negate it by inconsistent material from others. Certainly inconsistencies in what was obtained in the clinical interview and what he allegedly told the police or the authorities should be checked into in close detail during the second interview. Methods by which the patient handles this direct assault on his credibility should be noted and forms a part of his examination.

Clinical Evaluation of Amnesia

In many cases involving criminal behavior, especially homicide, the defendant often says he "can't remember what happened." The "not remembering" is usually a defensive reaction, but may represent true amnesia for the event.

Amnesia may be due to organic conditions (including tumor, stroke, heart attack, previous head trauma, arteriosclerosis or other degenerative or metabolic disorders causing brain dysfunction), alcoholic disorders, drug addiction or psychogenic factors, including repression, denial, hysterical forgetting, "true psychological blackout," later repression and lying (or malingering). The accurate determination of the nature of the amnesia often is difficult and occasionally impossible.

In order to attempt clarification of this confusing subject, we must first distinguish between amnesia and blackout. Amnesia is a forgetting at some later date events that occurred at a prior time that should have been remembered under ordinary circumstances. Forgetting may include preincident details, details of the incident and details following the incident. A blackout is not amnesia. It is a loss of, or alteration of, consciousness at a specific time for a specific duration of time, during which all conscious communication is obliterated. One will always have an amnesia for the period of the blackout; however, amnesia at some later times does not always mean there was a blackout of loss of consciousness at the time of the incident.

In the evaluation of amnesia the following steps are taken: first, one needs to take a careful history of the patient, including medical, psychological and developmental history, which include details of metabolic disorders, previous periods of unconsciousness or blackouts, head trauma, fractures, seizures, operations, familial illnesses, to rule out or rule in the possibility of organic etiology for either amnesia or blackout.

Next, one must conduct a complete physical examination of the individual for evidence of such organic problems. A careful psychiatric and psychological interview for the determination of psychodynamic conflicts, defense mechanisms and ego strengths, is necessary for other possible causes of amnesia, including hysteria, malingering and normal repression. It is quite common during an acute and violent outburst of rage culminating in the shooting or stabbing of another, that the perpetrator of the act will have an amnesia for the actual expression of his violent behavior.

This may be normal repression, an hysterical traumatic repression or a true blackout at the time of the murder. One means of determining the nature of this amnesia is by repeated careful interviews for evaluation of consistency of reporting, change in stories and addition of details.

Lie detector tests, Sodium Amytal interviews, hypnosis, prolonged and careful interviews, may help to overcome the repressive barrier and provide a more accurate evaluation of the state of amnesia.

In the event of conscious deception or psychoneurotic condition, the results of the sodium amytal interview may not be valid since one may continue the conscious deception while under the influence of amytal or may greatly exaggerate the situation at an unconscious level. Certainly the utterances of the patient under the influence of sodium amytal may not be admitted in evidence but can help the psychiatrist formulate his opinions which may be presented in evidence at trial. To aid in evaluating the credibility of statements of amnesia, the author frequently obtains a polygraph record designed to test whether the individual is lying about not remembering. If he passes the lie detector test, then a sodium amytal interview is conducted, using video tape recording to help uncover the lost or forgotten material.

Amnesia at the time of the incident does not preclude compeency to stand trial, even though the defendant may not be able effectively to cooperate with counsel in preparing a defense for the period of the crime. Also, amnesia does not mean lack of criminal responsibility in most jurisdictions. However, in some jurisdictions in which irresistible impulse is a part of the insanity test, such an impulsive shooting, stabbing or attack might be interpreted as part of an "insane" condition. Also, under the more liberal interpretations of the Currens Test and the American Law Institute Model Penal Code, the defendant may not have been able to "conform his conduct to the requirements of the law which he is alleged to have violated." In the military rules it may be said in many of these cases that the individual "could not adhere to the right" and thereby be found not guilty by reason of insanity.

Thus, the evaluation of amnesia may be an essential feature in the forensic psychiatric examination. Whenever the source of the forgetting is not determined accurately, the psychiatrist ought to so state. Also, it must be remembered that there are many causes for amnesia; mere forgetting is not necessarily related to competency or criminal responsibility.

Most interviews with defendants are not taped, though some psychiatrists prefer to record, verbatim, every psychiatric examination they conduct. Usually it is not necessary for such meticulous recording, since verbatim material is not necessary for substantiation of diagnoses. However, copious notes are usually taken by the psychiatrist during the initial interview and certain quotations or responses verbatim should be available for substantiation or corroboration of clinical impressions at time of trial.

The Forensic Psychiatric Report

The physician conducting the clinical interviews on a patient should prepare his report as follows: he should indicate name and age of the defendant, date and place of examination and who requested him to conduct the interview. He should also indicate length of time of interview(s) and what methods, tests or procedures were utilized in the examination. Also, what documents or statements were available to him in order to arrive at his conclusions, decisions and opinions. Primarily the psychiatrist relies upon his own clinical interview and psychological tests for arriving at his opinion, but he may have had access to other documents which form a partial basis for his conclusions.

Following this introductory material, the psychiatrist should then state in detail the present illness; i.e. present conditions leading up to the interview and examination, and detail as much as possible what the patient related about the instant offense. This part of the report should contain not only what the patient said but his responses, in affect and content, should be elaborated upon.

The next section usually deals with the past history, including developmental data, family history, early childhood memories and conflicts, educational, vocational and military history, marital and sexual history, medical and psychiatric history, all of which should contain relevant information to the current difficulty. These serve as building blocks of the past, a foundation for the current behavioral problems.

The next portion of the report usually contains a statement about current mental status examination, which is in detail and reflects aberrations of mood, affect, intelligence, orientation and ego strengths. Following is a subsection entitled "Diagnostic Impression" which contains the official nomenclature of the American Psychiatric Association, usually expanded in terms of manifestations and limitations of function.

The final section usually is entitled "summary and recommendations" or "summary and formulation." The summary is of the situation with appropriate formulation of current mental status and its relationship to the legal situation. That is, if he is pretrial, the conclusions apply to his mental ability to stand trial or his responsibility at the time of the alleged offense based on rules of criminal insanity for that particular jurisdiction. If he is in a presentence situation, the recommendations are for disposition including incarceration, hospitalization, psychotherapy or chemotherapy.

The recommendations need to be as specific as possible in order to aid the court in proper disposition. The report should be able to stand alone without elaboration, but often the psychiatrist is called to court to discuss in detail his findings, conclusions and recommendations. Often the court will not require psychiatric testimony and will rely on the report for advice and consultation.

The following two chapters will outline the role of the psychiatrist in consulting with referring attorneys in criminal cases and in presenting expert psychiatric testimony.

Chapter 4

PSYCHIATRIC CONSULTATION WITH REFERRING ATTORNEY IN PREPARATION FOR TRIAL

WHENEVER A PSYCHIATRIST is called by an attorney to examine a defendant in a criminal case, the psychiatrist should request of the attorney all available information including statements made by the defendant to police or authorities, any relevant past history or hospital material that the lawyer has obtained, as well as a statement of the charges and specific questions posed by the lawyer. This may be sent by mail prior to the initial examination for review by the examining psychiatrist. Depending on whether the attorney is present at time of initial interview, consultation will vary.

The initial interview of the defendant may take place in the psychiatrist's office if the defendant is on bail. However, in the event of nonbailable offenses or an indigent who is unable to post bail, the interview will need to take place in the prison. In many jurisdictions an independent psychiatrist may have difficulty getting into a prison to examine a defendant without a court order for such examination. In most jurisdictions homicide defendants will have a court-appointed attorney if the defendant is unable to afford private counsel. As part of the defense attorney's program, he may authorize independent psychiatric examination, evaluation and consultation. He will usually petition the court for such examination and request a court order be issued. The psychiatrist usually will need to take the court order with him to the prison in order to gain admittance for the interview.

Often the court will set a maximum limitation to the fee which it will pay the independent psychiatrist for his examination, evaluation and report. It is wise to have all these details spelled out prior to the examination. The court order and authorization are usually mailed by the attorney to the psychiatrist, with all the material necessary to conduct the initial interview.

Subsequent to the initial interview the doctor and lawyer may get together to discuss essential features of the problem. The psychiatrist has a duty to explain to the lawyer what he has found, based on specific disclosures by the patient and to give the lawyer, where possible, a diagnosis and tentative conclusion. Further, the doctor should present to the lawyer what other tests he would recommend, if any, and the reasons for these tests, with suggested or anticipated results. That is, what is the doctor looking for and how does he propose to find it? He should detail to the lawyer any inconsistencies he has found between the material given to the doctor by the lawyer and by the patient during the interview. He needs to have clear answers as to why these discrepancies or inconsistencies exist. He may suggest to the lawyer certain avenues of investigation that have emerged during the clinical interview which were not obtained by the lawyer during his interview. Certain family members or other acquaintances, or accomplices may need to be checked out, re-interviewed or examined by the psychiatrist.

The psychiatrist must be sure of the legal standard and criteria for insanity in the jurisdiction in which he is working; he must discuss these in detail with the lawyer with respect to the state of mind of the client/patient/defendant. If the psychiatrist feels that he has sufficient evidence to warrant an insanity defense, he should reveal this to the lawyer and indicate what this evidence is and how he proposes to present it under direct testimony and cross-examination. He must indicate what weak points exist in his formulation and where these may be bolstered and how they can be explained within reasonable medical certainty.

If the psychiatrist feels there is no basis for an insanity defense after the initial interview, he must explain in detail to the lawyer why he feels this is the case and what alternative considerations may be explored.

The psychiatrist who is called to examine a defendant must

work in close cooperation with the attorney for the accused. Prior to trial they must work as a team preparing the case on insanity, utilizing both legal and medical experience in formulating proper questions and anticipating cross-examination. Often, more time is spent consulting with counsel in preparing for a trial than is spent with the defendant himself. Counsel should not withhold information from his psychiatric expert, nor try to deceive him into coming to erroneous conclusions. This can only hurt at trial under precise cross-examination. The attorney who hopes to manipulate his expert witness into the belief that the defendant was insane at the time of the alleged crime, by not coming forward with bits of information or evidence which would refute that contention, is heading for trouble, since this information would likely be available to the prosecutor and would be brought out on cross-examination or during the case in rebuttal. To have the psychiatric witness surprised at trial is to have an unprepared witness who can only hurt the case for the attorney.

The foregoing is belabored because often an attorney is overzealously seeking a favorable verdict and does not wish to upset his psychiatrist's conclusions with material that could shed doubt on the firmness of his convictions. It is far better to present this material at pretrial conference and discuss it with the expert to determine whether it can fit into his conclusions, or whether indeed it negates the whole insanity defense. The latter is usually not the case and may be an exaggerated apprehension on the part of the attorney.

Following the initial psychiatric interview, any discrepancies or distortions between the defendant's version to the attorney and what he told the psychiatrist ought to be clarified. A variety of different stories spells trouble at trial. Many psychiatrists may feel put on the defensive if they are asked to change the wording of their statement or if they are asked to modify a statement so that it is presented in the best possible light for the client. Other psychiatrists recognize their role as part of a defense team whose goal is to obtain the best possible verdict for their client.

The optimal philosophy of preparing expert psychiatric testimony appears to be the following: the psychiatrist is called by the defense counsel to help him prepare the best possible defense within the limits of his medical expertise. He may advise counsel with respect to many factors including (1) the decision to have a jury trial, (2) the selection of a jury, (3) the kinds of questions that might be pertinent to ask prospective jurymen, (4) the best way of phrasing questions put to him on direct examination to obtain the most favorable responses, (5) which areas of inquiry to avoid on direct examination, and (6) advising counsel on cross-examination of other expert psychiatric witnesses. However, once the expert takes the witness stand and begins testifying, his allegiance belongs to the court, in the interests of justice. This may sound like an unattainable ideal, particularly when viewed from a practical point of view, but the court and jury will look to the expert witness as a neutral, scientific individual who is presenting his opinion in the light of impartiality, despite the fact that he may be called by one side or the other.

The defense counsel must recognize and understand this position from the outset and accept this role of his witness. He then realizes that he cannot depend completely upon the witness to present the testimony he needs for his verdict, but he must artfully bring this testimony to a clear and precise effect in the courtroom by use of his adversary role in direct and redirect examination.

This philosophy in preparing psychiatric experts will yield the most favorable testimony since it will keep the expert from feeling defensive and attacked by the prosecutor. He can only effectively be attacked if he feels that he has something to be attacked, that he is vulnerable, that he is an adversary. If he feels, however, that his testimony is in the best interest of honesty, truth, justice and integrity, he will think that it is his opinion and not himself that is under attack, especially where he recognizes that cross-examining counsel had a duty to question his testimony from all aspects in an attempt to invalidate it. The defense witness who becomes flustered and angry and feels that he is being attacked is a poor witness whose credibility will be questioned.

It is expected that effective cross-examination will bring out points that will tend to negate the effectiveness of the direct testimony. This should be expected, anticipated and allowed. If cross-examination is effective it is not the responsibility of the expert witness to stubbornly defend his statements. He need only support them from a scientific standpoint, where possible, and to corroborate his opinion based on his experience. The damage inflicted by good cross-examination can only be countered by equally effective redirect examination on those points made during cross-examination. Similarly, effective cross-examination of a psychiatric expert witness is an art which requires some skill, experience and often consultation with other psychiatric experts.

Case Example

Let us assume that an army sergeant with seventeen years of active duty, in full view of three eyewitnesses shot and killed another sergeant. Let us also suppose that the sergeant that was killed was a man known to have a violent temper, having beaten his wife on many occasions and having been brought before the MP's for reprimand because of domestic disruption. Further, the sergeant with the violent temper had been having several affairs with many of the wives on the base, and stayed out late, drinking, and had paid little attention to his wife, who befriended the defendant. Let us further assume that the sergeant who shot his peer had an affair with the victim's wife. Further, the victim had warned and threatened the defendant about staying away from his wife, or he, the victim, would kill the defendant. All of this was well known and documented by outside, objective observers.

On the day of the shooting the defendant heard that the victim was coming to "square things away" with him. In fear of his life, the defendant went home and got an old revolver which he had not used for several years and secreted it in his blouse "for protection." Instead of waiting for the confrontation, he went to the quarters of the victim in order to have the confrontation openly and "get it over with as soon as possible." Upstairs in the victim's room, the defendant and the victim decided to go "outside and settle this man to man." While walking down the stairs, however, the defendant found himself sandwiched between the victim and the victim's friend, a heavy, strong sergeant, who made threatening comments to the defendant on the way outside.

When outside, both the victim and his friend came at the defendant in a wedge, trapping him against a mound of earth. In fear and desperation the defendant pulled the gun from his blouse and warned both men to keep back. The victim's friend stopped and fell back but the victim said, "That little thing couldn't stop me." As the victim approached the defendant within several feet, without making an effort to stop, the defendant closed his eyes and pulled the trigger. From that time on, until he returned to the victim's quarters, the defendant remembered nothing. Eyewitnesses stated that the defendant pulled the trigger six times, emptying the contents of the gun into the victim. He stood over the fallen body, reloaded the revolver and emptied it once more into the victim's body, then walked to the victim's quarters and sat with the victim's wife until the MP's arrived.

On careful examination by both the defense attorney and the examining psychiatrist the story remained the same. Furthermore, the psychiatrist found on examination that the defendant never heard the shooting, neither did he remember the initial shooting, the reloading or the second shooting. He also indicated that he felt dazed and "not myself" until he got into the MP's car and felt the "cold steel of the handcuffs cutting my wrists."

The question here, of course, is what is the cause of the amnesia and what is the state of mind of the defendant at the time of the shooting. There is no question that the defendant caused the death of the victim by shooting, but, "is he guilty of murder?"

The defendant was born the middle of three children, having an older sister and a younger brother. He grew up in a rural area in the South, amidst poverty and financial difficulties. He recalls being teased and called embarrassing nicknames as a child. When talking about his relationship to his father and sister, saying that his father preferred his sister over him, he breaks spontaneously into tears. He grew up feeling unfairly treated by his father and crying often at the thought of this inequity. He also grew up fearing his father. He quit school early to go to work for economic reasons. As a youngster, however, he recalled being called "mother's baby" on many occasions by his friends. He did not date girls until he was nineteen or twenty, and did not have sexual intercourse until he was twenty-one years of age. He had a disturbing relationship with an American girl and vowed never to trust American girls after that. He was sent to Korea and began to live with Korean girls, whom he preferred. He has a long history of extramarital relationships, for which he says he always felt remorse, and which he always confessed to his wife, though he knew it would hurt her. He felt she had a right to know and she handled his confession with understanding. He frequently felt depressed and suicidal. He seemed sincere in the interviews and a reliable historian. There was some indication that he had feelings of inadequacy as a male, as manifested by his frequent extramarital activities, his past history of inadequate functioning with other boys and his close relationship to his mother, which prevented his emancipating himself as early as his peers.

Because of the discrepancy in his memory and the seriousness of the crime, a sodium amytal interview was conducted to determine whether the amnesia was based on a subsequent repression or forgetting after the act, or based on a "blackout" at the time of the shooting. Many people find it psychologically easier to handle the period subsequent to a killing by repressing that fact and not remembering details. This is often quite normal. However, there are people who have actual blackouts or altered states of consciousness at the time of the crimes which are naturally not remembered because the individual was not fully conscious at the significant time.

The sodium amytal interview also revealed a consistency in the defendant's statements to both the attorney and to the psychiatrist under clinical conditions. He was still unable to recall completely the events which occurred on the day of the shooting, but did recall shooting the victim six times, rather than merely squeezing the trigger and then forgetting. He was unable to recall reloading or the subsequent shooting of six bullets. Other factors learned under sodium amytal included an elaboration of his feelings of inadequacy as a male and an emergence of his latent homosexual fears.

The conclusion of the examining psychiatrist after the sodium amytal interview was that the defendant had indeed suffered a blackout at the time of the shooting, not a complete loss of consciousness, but an altered state of consciousness based on homosexual panic (which often leads to an acute paranoid schizophrenic reaction or break with reality). This reaction may represent a temporary psychotic condition, rendering a person completely unable to "adhere to the right." In this sense the defendant's condition met the requirements of legal insanity under the military rules (though not in Mc-Naghten's jurisdictions) rendering testimony to this effect most pertinent at his court-martial.

Although utterances made under the influence of sodium amytal are inadmissible at trial, evidence of the test may be used to substantiate or corroborate other impressions gained by the psychiatrist in formulating his opinion, as may an X ray or psychological tests elaborate on other clinical material. In this case the amytal interview was imperative. Its results were significant in the formulation of a diagnosis that at the time of the shooting the defendant's state of mind rendered him unable to adhere to the right.*

In preparing this case for trial, counsel must be certain that the psychiatrist is convinced of his impression, his diagnosis and his conclusions. Defense counsel must play devil's advocate in

---

* For a more comprehensive discussion of the sodium amytal test and other similar tests, please see Chapter 6.

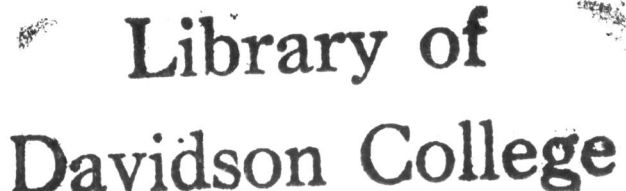

asking questions which could be anticipated on cross-examination to prepare the witness for that phase of his examination. Certainly, the proper answers to questions which would otherwise tend to destroy his direct testimony would leave the cross-examining attorney short of his desired goal. The testimony must be rehearsed prior to the trial. This dry run should include qualifying the expert, direct testimony and anticipated cross-examination. The responses by the witness will give defense counsel a chance to formulate questions for redirect examination, should it be deemed necessary.

Let us now take this case through a dry run. After the witness is sworn and identified the initial questions asked are those which would qualify him as an expert in his profession and include where he was trained, what extra training he may have had, his medical school and whether it is accredited, his internship and residency training and what the residency included. This is to be followed by a statement of licensure after which the following are included: membership in various national medical and psychiatric organizations, with offices held; whether the individual is board-certified by the American Board of Psychiatry and Neurology and therefore entitled Diplomate in Psychiatry and Neurology, with certificate (asked only if he is). This certification requires successful completion of a number of examinations and only about one third of psychiatrists are so certified. If the psychiatrist has presented papers at national meetings or published papers that would be significant to the case, these should be elaborated upon. Any positions that he holds in teaching, research and service to the community should also be presented. Finally, the expert's experience in evaluating and treating people involved in criminal matters and his experience in testifying as an expert and for whom.

The purpose of the presentation of qualifications is twofold: first, a factual documentation on which the court bases its acceptance of the witness; second, its effect on the court and the jury. That is, if the expert is well qualified with a number of well-recognized positions and honors, the credibility of his conclusions and supporting testimony is enhanced.

The next question should be phrased to enable the witness to explain the facts and circumstances of his examination of the defendant. The doctor should be asked what the examination consisted of and what he learned from it. This will usually allow the expert witness to present in narrative summary what the patient told him at the time of the examination. This may be as long and as detailed a narrative as is appropriate and as desired by the witness-psychiatrist. The witness also should be asked what statements, documents or other materials were used in his examination and in reaching his conclusions. All facets of the doctor's examination and evaluation should be included and related to the court: interviews with the defendant's family, including parents, sisters, brothers, spouse, MP's/police officers, medical records, if available, and discussions with counsel. Since psychological tests are usually prepared on cases of this nature, they will be discussed and elaborated upon from the standpoint of aid to the psychiatrist in reaching his conclusion.

The sodium amytal interview should be approached during direct examination by asking the psychiatrist whether other tests were conducted prior to reaching his conclusion and diagnosis. Although witnesses cannot testify as to what was said verbatim under the influence of sodium amytal, certainly consistencies, corroborations or inconsistencies may be presented adjunctively to the conclusionary statements reached by the psychiatrist in making his evaluation. This material should be presented in terms of and as an adjunctive test for the determination of whether or not the loss of memory at the time of the shooting was a true amnesia. The testimony concerning the verity of the amnesic condition, an altered state of consciousness, at the time of the shooting is a conclusion based on two criteria: (a) the use of sodium amytal and (b) the psychiatrist's interpretation of the abreaction of the patient, which indicated to him that the defendant's response to the medication was spontaneous. It should be noted that under sodium amytal some people can consciously deceive and continue a prevarication that was initiated in clinical examination. Others may grossly exaggerate the circumstances while having an unusual reaction to the sodium amytal.

The counselor on direct examination of the expert may proceed as follows.

Q. Doctor, based on your clinical examination of the patient and all the adjunctive tests and materials that you studied, have you arrived at a conclusion as to a diagnosis of the defendant?
A. Yes
Q. What is your diagnosis?
A. The diagnosis is chronic depressive reaction with schizoid personality adjustment, manifested by feelings of inadequacy and mistrust for others, occasional bizarre and unusual behavior with response to internal rather than external reality.
Q. Doctor, is this a recognized mental illness, disease or derangement?
A. Yes
Q. Doctor, do you have an opinion as to the state of mind of the defendant at the time of the shooting on (date)?
A. Yes
Q. What is your opinion as to that diagnosis?
A. It is my opinion that on that date at the time of the shooting, he was suffering from an altered state of consciousness due to an acute psychotic reaction precipitated by homosexual panic under acute stress by his feeling that his life was being threatened. His diagnosis of schizoid personality and depressive reaction was such that it is likely under proper and sufficient stress, he could break down to an acute psychotic reaction.
Q. Doctor, at the time of the shooting, then, while under the acute psychotic reaction, do you have an opinion as to whether or not his mental condition prevented him from knowing the difference between right and wrong?
A. Yes
Q. What is that opinion?
A. It would be improbable or unlikely for him to consider the difference between right and wrong at the time of his acute psychotic reaction or break with reality.
Q. Doctor, on the basis of your examination and with the diag-

Consultation With Referring Attorney

nosis of acute psychoatic reaction, do you have an opinion as to whether or not the defendant at the time of the shooting was able to adhere to the right?
A. Yes
Q. What is that opinion?
A. Based on this man's diagnosis and his mental condition of acute psychotic reaction at the time of the shooting, it is my opinion that he was unable to adhere to the right.

Cross-Examination

The cross-examination of this type of defense lends itself to many standard questions, usually asked of the witness. They may be summarized as follows.

Q. Doctor, when did you first examine the defendant?
A. (date)
Q. Doctor, how long is that after the shooting took place?
A. About six months
Q. And you did not see the defendant prior to that time?
A. No
Q. How long did you spend with the defendant in total?
A. Five to six hours
Q. Do you feel you know the defendant well enough to present expert psychiatric testimony today?
A. Yes
Q. How long do you usually spend examining defendants prior to testifying in court?
A. Usually between five to ten hours but it varies with the problem and the special tests required.
Q. Doctor, isn't it true that your opinion is based primarily on what the defendant told you?
A. My opinion is based in part on what the defendant told me but I took into account other documents, other corroborating evidence.
Q. Then what you are telling us is merely what the defendant has stated to you and you are repeating back to us, isn't that so, Doctor?
A. Not entirely, since my opinion is based not so much on the

content of what he has told me but on his affective responses while he is presenting the material. Thus, I am aware of his emotional as well as intellectual responses to my questions. Also, I did a sodium amytal interview in which he reacted spontaneously; reactions which were not contrived responses. That is to say, under the maximal effect of the amytal, his responses were spontaneous, without consideration or calculation.

Q. But now, doctor, aren't they all statements that come from the defendant without corroboration from anyone else?

A. Yes, in a sense, in the sodium amytal interview all the statements come from the defendant; however, unlike normal interviews which contain conscious statements, these were spontaneous and without undue consideration.

Q. Could he lie under the influence of sodium amytal?

A. Yes

Q. Now doctor, you testified that it was your opinion that he was suffering from an acute psychotic reaction at the time of the shooting. How do you know that?

A. My opinion is based on my examinations of the defendant and the data I have collected.

Q. Well doctor, that is your opinion only, isn't that right? You really don't know that he was suffering from this illness at the time because you were not there, isn't that right, doctor?

A. Yes, that is right. I do not know with absolute certainty because I was not present. But I do have an opinion based on reasonable medical certainty.

Q. Isn't it possible, doctor, that the defendant could have fabricated this "amnesia?"

A. Yes, but it is not likely that he did so.

Q. But it is possible, is it not, that he could have conveniently "forgotten," as many defendants do after such a traumatic episode?

A. Yes, it is possible.

Q. Now, doctor, did you speak to any of the eyewitnesses or examine their statements or reports about the defendant's state of mind at the time of the shooting?

A. No, I did not examine their statements nor did I interview them.
Q. Then no one described him as having a glazed look or looking crazy or not being himself?
A. That's correct.
Q. Do you think it would have been helpful, doctor, if you had gotten an eyewitness account of his state of mind, rather than relying on your opinion alone, which was six months after the shooting?
A. It is sometimes helpful to obtain the statements of eyewitnesses about appearances of defendants but not always so.
Q. Do you think it would have been helpful in this case?
A. It may have been.
Q. Then your sources of information were incomplete, were they not?
A. They were in that sense.
Q. Now doctor, where else has your source of information been incomplete so that you arrived at your conclusion with insufficient information?
A. I don't feel that my sources were incomplete sufficiently to jeopardize my conclusions or my opinion.
Q. Now doctor, were you aware that the defendant was having a sexual affair with the victim's wife?
A. Yes
Q. Isn't it possible, doctor, that he shot the victim to get him out of the way so he could have his wife?
A. It is possible, but I don't feel it was the case here.
Q. Now doctor, do you have any prior history of the defendant's having an acute psychotic break such as the one you describe his having conveniently at the time of the shooting?
A. No
Q. Doctor, you testified that it was your opinion that at the time of the shooting it was improbable or unlikely for him to consider the difference between right and wrong. Do you have an opinion whether at that time he knew what he was doing was wrong?
A. No

Q. How did the amytal test do that?
A. His responses were spontaneous and supported a repression of or amnesia for the events that occurred while he was psychotic.
Q. Is it possible the amnesia was not real but the defendant deceived you?
A. It is possible but not likely.

On redirect examination the points to pick up are the validity of the examination, including the sodium amytal interview which renders the witness certain of his diagnosis, and his impression and conclusion about insanity at the time of the offense. Also stress the conclusions as to treatment and disposition to impress upon the jury/court that the defendant will not be going "scot-free" to "kill again." Rather, he will be treated or evaluated and confined until the doctors feel he is sufficiently safe to be treated as an outpatient, and will not pose a threat or danger to others.

Thus, the aim of direct testimony is to present as credible a statement about the defendant's state of mind at the time of the offense as possible, with sincere conviction on the part of the witness that this is not only his opinion but a valid conclusion which is the most plausible alternative to consider. On the other hand, the function of the cross-examination is to destroy this credibility and to attempt to present other alternatives which could be tendered just as readily.

Chapter 5

THE PSYCHIATRIST IN THE COURTROOM

IN ORDER FOR THE PSYCHIATRIST to work effectively in the legal arena, he must be aware of the rules of the game, the players and their roles and special procedures relating to his work. In the first place the psychiatrist must understand that a trial is an adversary procedure in which two sides oppose each other, whether it be a criminal trial, a civil trial, a hearing or a special legal procedure. The two sides are represented by counsel (lawyers) who are well trained in the rules of the game. As moderator or arbitrator, a judge or a master rules on all aspects of the trial. He decides all points of contention (often called objections) and settles disputes within the major arena. There are rules of evidence that must be followed and it is up to the judge to referee when these rules are broken.

The psychiatrist may be called in to testify as an expert witness by one side or the other, or by the court. What the psychiatrist must understand is that it doesn't really matter which side initially calls him. Once he is sworn in as an expert witness, his allegiance is only to the court, not to the attorney or patient or client/defendant.

Too often we see psychiatrists who are on the defensive under cross-examination because their testimony is attacked logically, clearly and sometimes emotionally by the opposing attorney. It must be understood that when a psychiatrist undertakes to examine a client, if his evaluation is not consistent with the needs of the attorney calling him he most likely will not testify. If, however, he indicates that his testimony will be helpful to the side that has retained him, he will be called to the stand. One cannot expect 100 percent correlation of psychiatric testimony to the requirements of the side calling him, in all cases. Certainly there will be many cases in which the evaluation is a difficult one, bordering on a close decision.

Just as in clinical case conferences where there is room for differential diagnoses, there is also room for disagreement in the courtroom. Practitioners of psychiatry, and especially those who are willing to expose their knowledge and experience to critical evaluation (a situation which does not ordinarily occur in private practice) must expect alternative views of their findings to be presented. Thus, different psychiatrists may present varying opinions, reflecting the reality that psychiatry is not an exact science and cannot be expected to perform as such.

Preparation of Psychiatric Evidence

The forensic psychiatrist preparing his testimony must take into consideration as many facts and as much information as is available to him. As stressed in previous chapters, it is not sufficient for him merely to do a good psychiatric examination. He must also have at his disposal a variety of documents: previous records, statements or confessions made by the patient or defendant at the time of the offense, etc.

In one case the author testified regarding the suppression of a confession because the individual was intellectually inferior and psychotic at the time he made the confession and was unable intelligently to waive his rights, have a lawyer present or to remain silent. When asked if the policemen taking the confession had been interviewed (men who were present at the time) the reply was "No," since this was not a usual part of the examination. The judge and the district attorney of course were surprised, since here was provided an opportunity to talk to the people who were present at the time in question, ones that could provide further information.

It is now a regular part of the author's comprehensive forensic evaluation to include the opinion of any policemen who had the opportunity of seeing the defendant at a time nearer to the crime. This is so especially when the testimony refers to a mental state at some previous time to examination and not only to competency at the time of the interview.

One other instance that comes to mind about the collection of comprehensive information occurred when several colleagues and the author testified in a case in another country. The others had examined the defendant extensively but had no access to, nor did they care to have access to, the confession or the opinions of other people who were present at the time the crime was committed. The author insisted that this information be made available as part of a comprehensive examination. One of the psychiatrists who had experience in legal matters indicated that that was not important; that all he cared to present was the psychiatric examination that he had conducted on the defendant, several months after the crime. The author was reprimanded for trying to "act like a lawyer." He insisted that a psychiatrist is a tool of the law and can present only the psychiatric examination. He said we ought to let the law and the judges use the other data as they see fit.

However, the author feels that any opinion about mental state at some previous time cannot be determined solely on the basis of an examination several months or years later. It must include other information relevant to the client's mental state at that time, in addition to his own description.

Psychiatric Testimony

Since the direct examination is usually rehearsed in a pretrial conference, the expert witness should have no difficulty with that part of his testimony. However, cross-examination by a bright, well-trained, perceptive attorney can prove to be difficult and disconcerting to the expert who is not used to having his medical word challenged. There is no room for arrogance or conceit in the courtroom. There is only room for honest opinion based on sound examination and clinical experience.

Just as in training, a supervisor may question the psychiatric resident's initial diagnosis and evaluation of a patient, so it is with the cross-examining attorney. He may not know as much about the patient or about psychiatry as the expert, but you can be sure he will try to present evidence that might lead to a different diagnosis. Usually, he will have had the consultation of another psychiatrist and may even have another psychiatrist in the courtroom, aiding him in his questioning. The important thing to remember is that the psychiatrist is not on trial, and neither are his opinions. His opinions must be presented as just this; they are not facts.

In most instances the cross-examining attorney is not sufficiently astute to threaten the expert, either logically or emotionally. Some who may feel inadequate in their attack on the expert's testimony, may resort to trickery in order to fluster the witness, stimulating him to argue, become upset, angry, embarrassed, frightened and certainly anxious. As soon as the expert resorts to a defensive attitude, a feeling that he must protect his integrity and defend his word, he is subject to weakness in his presentation.

If the cross-examining attorney finds logical evidence and good medical thinking to attack the expert's testimony, it behooves the psychiatrist to reconsider his original opinion. The passive psychiatrist may back down and change his opinion on the stand. This, of course, is what the cross-examining attorney intends the witness to do. Or, the psychiatrist will not change his opinion for fear of professional criticism and internal feelings of incompetency, but will so contradict himself and weaken his testimony as to make it totally ineffective.

Whereas rigidity on the stand or stubbornness cannot be advocated, the following points are stressed. (1) The expert should come dressed appropriately for his part in this game. This usually means a conservative suit, not a flashy sports jacket. On hot days it may be permissible, on approval of the judge, to remove one's jacket, but this usually is not done in modern, air-conditioned courtrooms. (2) The psychiatrist should sit straight and dignified, without slouching or leaning in an awkward position. There is nothing more offensive to a lay jury than to see a psychiatrist or a physician on the stand attempting to handle his anxiety by assuming a flamboyant air. Cockiness can never replace self-assuredness, and a casual attitude with flippancy must never substitute for calmness and composure.

In all cases the psychiatrist must be prepared as thoroughly as possible to present his testimony and his opinions, anticipating the kinds of questions that might tend to weaken it. If one can anticipate accurately in the cross-examination, he is much the better and often ahead of the game, just as he was in medical school when he could anticipate correctly the questions to be asked on an exam. To be rigid and stubborn is to be insecure; flexibility without fragility is the key.

There is nothing more pitiful than to see a leading member of the community, a distinguished physician, brought to his knees under cross-examination because he is ill prepared and not in touch with current psychiatric principles. There are many legal tricks that the cross-examining attorney uses and the expert should be aware of these "tricks" and how to handle them.

Many questions are asked by the cross-examining attorney that are meant to trick or trap the expert into being inconsistent or even contradictory. It is often difficult, after hours of cross-examination, to remember every detail that one has said. One may be tripped up, and it is not unlikely that he will be. The point is not to get flustered if this happens. It need not discredit one's whole testimony, as the attorney would wish to convey to the jury.

A psychiatrist is as liable to err as anyone else. Feelings of omnipotence and omniscience should be left in the office, along with narcissism. Being human is often very appealing to the human lay jurors. One thing that can be done if the question is a trick one is to ask the lawyer to repeat it, or pause to give the other attorney a chance to object to it. If there is any question about clarifying an answer, requesting a clarification from the judge is usually granted and may be very important. The judge is the boss: he can ask questions, he can cross-examine, he can make decisions that the lawyers do not challenge until later. If the witness feels that the cross-examining attorney is arguing or getting emotional or upset, or being unfair in any way, he should feel free to point this out to the judge.

Another point to remember is that if psychiatric testimony is modified under cross-examination, it is not the witness' responsibility to undo the modification. This is the responsibility of the attorney calling his expert. He is running his case and it is up to him to ask the questions, make the points, using expert testimony to do so, just as the cross-examining attorney will use the expert's testimony to discredit his opponent's case.

The psychiatrist in court is the tool of the court and is used as such. The first time one testifies can be a most anxiety-provoking experience. Anxiety will be one's worst enemy. The psychiatrist's anxiety will often trip him up and stimulate him to say something he had no intention of saying, especially under cross-examination. There are many methods the psychiatrist may use in dealing with a difficult cross-examination. Some have advocated the psychiatrist consider the opposing attorney as a sick patient, at whom the doctor rarely, if ever, gets angry or flustered, but handles with dispatch and expertise, based on clinical experience. One has even suggested that the psychiatrist consider the attorney a paranoid schizophrenic who will ask "crazy questions" the answers to which are much easier. The author's personal feeling is that this kind of approach may work only occasionally, and is certainly not fair either to the psychiatrist, the attorney or the patient/client. If one takes the experience in its entirety and looks at it from a comprehensive point of view, the following is much more appropriate and relevant.

Just as the psychiatrist must do his homework before going to court, exposing his knowledge (or lack of it) to the world, so must the attorney. The bright, well-prepared attorney is a pleasure to observe. The poorly prepared one, by contrast, may look ridiculous. Whereas we may hope that our opposing attorney has not done his homework and lets us off quite easily, it really is not fair, for the most is not gained from our testimony.

If the opposing counsel is well prepared and bright, he may actually enhance our testimony by raising points that we had not considered. The psychiatrist must remember that he is not on trial, neither are his evaluative techniques, nor his expertise. The disciplines of law and of psychiatry both may stimulate a narrowness in the individual and his viewpoint. How much greater was our general horizon as freshmen in college than as seniors in medical school. How much narrower have our frames of reference become after psychiatric residency. Experience may be greater but perspective narrows. The law, on the other hand, as narrow as it may be to its own practitioners, brings to the psychiatrist an exposure to a different way of thinking.

It is always a pleasure to respond to a bright, perceptive and well-prepared cross-examining attorney. True, he may attack my testimony and weaken it, or even point up where my conclusions are not soundly based on my observations, but one must keep an open mind and a humble approach.

We must recognize that we only do the best we can with the time we have alloted for the examination and with the material we have available. It is possible that the other side has other evidence or material that we had not considered. Often the question will run, "Now doctor if you know that Mr. Jones also participated in homosexual activities, would that change your opinion or your diagnosis?" Supposing we had not been availed of this information, would it change our diagnosis? It might enhance our diagnosis, it might support it, it might fit in as a piece of the puzzle we found missing. Or, it might change our evaluation entirely, and we would have to do a complete reevaluation of the individual and his case, based on the new material gained at time of trial. This, of course, would be most unusual, and is used only as an extreme example to point out the possibilities that exist.

If the cross-examining attorney cannot discredit the testimony of the psychiatrist, he may attempt to discredit the integrity of the psychiatrist. For example, the question is asked, "Now, doctor, how much are you getting paid for testifying today?" This sounds like a very demeaning question. After all, we never discuss money. Money is degrading and talk of it should not be heard in such hallowed halls as a courtroom. However, the question is often asked; it is asked primarily if the cross-examining attorney has failed or feels that he has failed to gain points with his relevant questioning.

The answer, of course, is that we are getting paid nothing to testify. We are getting paid for our time as we would if we were to spend it in our offices or anywhere else, taking care of professional matters. After all, a professional is entitled to a professional fee. One would not expect us to work for nothing. One does not have to be defensive about this, only realistic. One example will illustrate how this question was handled recently by an experienced forensic psychiatrist who had been under cross-examination for four hours without successful attack on his testimony. He replied to the question, "That all depends on how long you keep me here." This answer was designed to relieve the tension, bring humor to the courtroom and to make the cross-examining attorney look foolish for his "wasting time on trivial questions." It was also a relevant answer because the expert indicated that he was being paid for his time and not for his testimony.

Some Notes on Fees

Because all examinations for lawyers involve not only the time spent with the patient/client/defendant, but also time spent with counsel and time preparing a proper and significant report, the author usually advises that *initial* examinations for any legal purpose be at the rate of 25 percent to 50 percent above the usual hourly rate charged for therapy. Any time spent with the attorney in discussing his case should be billed, as should all time spent in reading pages of testimony and preparing a report. It is here we can learn from our legal colleagues, since they usually collect a retainer in advance, to protect their interests. This is extremely important, especially in criminal cases for, if the defendant is convicted and sent to prison, there may be no fee forthcoming. It is a change from our usual method of sending bills and collecting fees at some later date, and not offending our patients by discussing collection of money in advance or even personally.

Often we resort to the mails or to a secretary to collect the money, rather than taking it ourselves. This need not be the case.

Special procedures such as sodium amytal interviews, or court appearances should be billed at a higher fee. One can never predict the length of time he will be in court, nor the length of time it would take for a special procedure away from his office. For this reason, a half-day or daily fee is charged rather than an hourly one. This is to account for the inconvenience of rescheduling patients, being placed on last minute notice and traveling some distance to court or another office. It is also appropriate because the subspecialty of forensic psychiatry demands further specialized training and the preparation and presentation of adequate testimony is a special procedure within psychiatry.

Often the lawyer will wish the psychiatrist to be in court for several days to observe witnesses and to aid the attorney in his cross-examination of other psychiatrists, and of other witnesses. In that case a daily rate should be charged and should be discussed with the attorney prior to participation. It is often advisable in prolonged and expensive cases to receive a retainer for half the anticipated amount before proceeding.

Again, we are not paid for our services, but for our time. In the same way, in testifying to a civil case of trauma or negligence, where a large award may be granted, the psychiatrist never testifies on contingency; i.e. he is paid his usual fee for his time, irrespective of the outcome of the case. His services are not contingent upon the client receiving a large monetary award.

Teaching Function of Expert Testimony

One of the most important functions we have as expert witnesses is to teach others what we have learned. We are not on the stand to defend our abilities, our talents or our profession; we are there only to share with the law, especially the judge and jury, the benefits of our experience and training in a highly flexible discipline called psychiatry. Having been both a consultee and a consultant in psychiatry, i.e. a student and a teacher, it is safe to say that often more is learned as a consultant when teaching than as a consultee (when learning from my teacher). So it is true on the stand, as an expert witness, we are there to teach but we must also learn. We may learn through good cross-examination or by sitting in court and hearing other testimony on the matter not obtained during clinical examination.

We have no special allegiance in court to the defendant or patient just because he is paying us. Our only allegiance on the witness stand is to the court. This is usually made very clear to the lawyers who call me into court, and often they are disconcerted when they find that my testimony is modified under perceptive and pointed cross-examination. It is modified but not necessarily weakened because it is advantageous to appear reasonable and flexible rather than rigid and defensive on the stand.

It is enlightening to work with attorneys who have shown diligence and perception in cases involving psychiatric problems and are able to utilize their talents to bring the points into focus. Instead of feeling threatened and upset or angry at an attorney who raises important and significant questions which may weaken our testimony, we should react positively as we learn more about our patient and our own role with him in his legal situation.

In summary, we are consultants on the witness stand; we are experts; we are not decision-makers or fact-finders. Realization of this role should allay much anxiety in the uninitiated psychiatric expert.

The Hypothetical Question

One of the most disconcerting and anxiety-provoking aspects of presenting expert testimony for the psychiatrist is the "hypothetical question." Many colleagues ask me, "What do I do when they ask me the hypothetical?" The hypothetical question is really a very simple construct. It is the reiteration of all the relevant facts that have gone into evidence thus far that the psychiatrist has not been in court to hear, or evidence that will subsequently be introduced. It always begins with the words: "Now doctor, assume that . . ." and then a repeat of the pertinent points that have been raised in evidence or will be raised. These are the facts on which the question is based and the answer is sought.

The psychiatrist has most of these facts before he gets into the courtroom, if he has done his homework and has had access to the materials necessary for proper forensic evaluation. Having had access to most of the information, he may hear little or nothing new in the hypothetical and will give his opinion as rehearsed. Most often the hypothetical will be asked by the attorney calling the psychiatrist to testify and will have been gone over in a pretrial conference. If new facts are introduced in a hypothetical by cross-examining attorney, the witness must evaluate his opinion in light of the new evidence.

Communication

Another point that must be mentioned here is the use of language. The psychiatrist who is narrowed by his training, begins to use the language of his discipline, feels a certain special quality about it and may even feel a little pompous about its use, since he knows what the words mean and others may not. There is no place for this type of language or mal-communication in the courtroom. Proper English is necessary because the primary purpose we have in a courtroom is to communicate, and if we use language that is not understood, we have failed in our purpose. Simple, direct statements spoken in clear tones while facing the jury or the judge and talking to them, and not at them, is advisable.

An example will illustrate several points: The author was called into a military case as the "expert from the big city," testifying in behalf of a young man who had deserted his camp. There was every indication that he was psychotic at the time, and this was presented in a clear, straightforward manner, with subsequent poor cross-examination. The military psychiatrist who had less time to examine the defendant found that he was not psychotic, and did not feel he was psychotic at the time of his act. He sat in the middle of the courtroom (as is the custom in the military) surrounded by defense on one side and prosecution on the other, while facing the court of officers. He spoke with his head down, mumbled his words, and seemed to be awed by his disagreement with the "expert from the big city." He was of no value to his side, nor to the determination, since very few could hear him, and others must have felt, as the author did, that he was unsure of what he was saying.

This may sound like forensic psychiatric testimony needs to be rehearsed and practiced; that psychiatrists must have a flamboyant air and be "on stage" while in the witness chair. This is not the case entirely, but certainly communication is not limited to words alone. It includes such factors as affect, appearance, demeanor, confidence, all of which go to the credibility of the testimony. Remember, there are rules to follow and there are roles to play. If one is to play the role he should play it as well as possible. To the layman it may seem a harsh way of promoting justice and truth, but consider the difference in talent and ability of various attorneys. Many a case is won or lost on the ability and the presentation of the attorney, rather than on the validity of his case. Logic and reason are only the essence of what is needed to be communicated. The vehicle by which this is communicated to the court is also extremely significant. The essence becomes lost if the vehicle breaks down and never reaches its destination.

To sum up, the attitude of the psychiatrist as expert witness should be a dignified one with the purpose of teaching or sharing information in the most appropriate and expressive manner, while learning from the other participants. The courtroom is no place to change the law or try and present the ideal situation. The psychiatrist is the guest in the house of the law and must comport himself as such, or he should not accept the invitation to be there.

Chapter 6

PSYCHIATRIC INVOLVEMENT IN THE SEARCH FOR TRUTH

THE AVOWED PURPOSE of any legal proceeding primarily is to ascertain the truth of the matter and to render proper justice. The ideal concept of truth, however, is an elusive abstract not always definable in practical terms. In our adversary approach to judicial proceedings the truth of a man's statements and the validity of his testimony may need to be determined tangentially and indirectly.

Contrary to popularly held superstitious and mythical beliefs, a man's mind; i.e. his thoughts and intents, cannot be "read" by others. Current research in extrasensory perception and mental telepathy has not disproved this axiom. Since the law must ascertain a man's intent in relation to his behavior in order properly to carry out its function, it has resorted to various means to learn the truth of one's statements and to gain confessions from accused individuals.

Legal history is replete with cases of torture and brutality imposed upon accused individuals to "get them to confess." The ancient Romans knew that *in vino veritas* and used such drugs as opium, modragora, hemp, carbon dioxide and alcohol to facilitate confessions. Later, peyote was used by Mexican Indians for the same purpose. In the early twentieth century, T. S. House, an American anesthesiologist, stumped the country proclaiming the advantages scopolamine had in extracting confessions, and he coined the term "truth serum." Since then, other forms of "truth sera" such as sodium pentothal and sodium amytal have been used to determine the veracity of statements and to obtain confessions.

Originally published in the *American Bar Ass'n Journal*, March, 1966, Vol. 52, No. 3, p. 251.

This scientific wedge in the door to psychological means of approaching the truth in law was driven further by the introduction of polygraph machines, called lie detectors; later, hypnosis and psychiatric interviews were instituted for similar uses. Most recently, projective psychological testing has been called upon by the law to aid in the determination of truth.

The increasing utilization of psychiatrists and psychiatric techniques in the law has raised a number of ethical and legal issues. Psychiatric interviews, psychological tests, evaluation under hypnosis, so-called lie detector tests and truth serum examinations have all been used to help determine the truthfulness of statements, the validity of confessions, the nature of memory loss (e.g. amnesia, malingering) and the mental responsibility of criminal defendants.

There are many historical, sociological, legal, scientific and practical reasons why these techniques have become involved in the complexities of our judicial system. Critics often have asked whether psychiatrists and psychologists ought to intrude into this delicate area. Such issues as limitation of freedom and infringement of constitutional rights have been presented as well as the ethical problems involving confidentiality and the medical duty to "do no harm."

By involving himself in this situation and offering his services to the community and legal agencies, the psychiatrist has indeed tread upon dangerous and hostile ground. He has risked and received open censure for his intrusion and yet has remained in the interest of promoting justice and in the hope of furthering general knowledge and understanding of human behavior.

Generally, the law has been quite suspicious of the psychiatric intruder and has dealt with him as such. His science has been termed infantile and his findings subjected to hostile criticism. Courts generally have felt that psychiatry has offered little to the precision required by the law. Psychiatric testimony often has been given little weight as expert testimony and has been termed of no greater value than direct observation by laymen.

When psychiatrists responded to these criticisms and began sharpening their approach by utilizing more precise methods of evaluation, the courts reacted by declaring these methods an infringement of constitutional safeguards and refused to admit, directly, testimony gained by use of such means.

The principal legal criticisms of these scientific tests or methods fall into three general categories: (a) their constitutionality, (b) their scientific standing and (c) their invasion of the province of the jury.[1] The outstanding comments allude to the denial or limitation of the constitutional safeguards of due process of law when such scientific tests are employed.

Guttmacher advances the proposition that, "Paramount among the principles of judicial procedure, established by the history of due process, are the facts that the procedure must be adversary and not inquisitorial and that the accused is at all times a 'party' to the trial and must be present in criminal proceedings at all times. When these devices for exploring the unconscious are employed, the defendant is in truth present in body only, but not in mind."[2]

Szasz carries this theme further: "The expanding use of psychiatric intervention in the enforcement of the criminal law has, in my opinion, steadily diminished our constitutional liberties. The recent practice of pretrial psychiatric examination of defendants on the order of the court and against the wishes of the accused, promised to effectively nullify some of our most important constitutional rights, namely, the right to a speedy trial and the right, in the words of Louis D. Brandeis, 'to be let alone.'"[3]

The question of reliability of these scientific and psychiatric tests is a very real one. Subjective interpretation of "objective" findings is always open to error and to the degree of variability in the examiners. Guttmacher indicates, "None of these tests produces results automatically. The tests must be administered with scrupulous objectivity and the results skillfully analyzed and scrutinized. Their degree of reliability is in no small measure dependent upon the testor."[2]

Courts have rejected the results of lie detector tests when offered in evidence for purpose of establishing guilt or innocence of one accused of crime. The reasons given are usually that the lie detector test has not as yet attained scientific acceptance as a reliable and accurate measure of ascertaining truth or deception.*

As stated succinctly by a recent Kansas decision:

> There is no persuasive analogy here with such tests as fingerprinting which have a strictly physical basis, clearly demonstrable. It is not contended that the lie detector measures or weighs the important psychological factors. Many innocent but highly sensitive persons would undoubtedly show unfavorable physical reactions, while many guilty persons of heightened or less sensitive spirit, would register no physical indication of falsification. This the trained operators, of course, understand and proceed upon the basis of the large percentage of error. But it seems quite too subtle a task of evaluation to impose upon an untrained jury.[5]

Even if the lie detector test does attain scientific acceptance, the constitutionality of evidence so obtained would still be in issue.

The results of truth serum examination and hypnosis occupy the same position in the court decisions.

> These devices are unlike the science of handwriting, fingerprinting or X ray, which reflect demonstrable physical facts that require no complicated interpretation predicated upon the hazards of unknown individual emotional differences, which may and often do result in erroneous conclusions. Although narcoanalysis in general and sodium pentothal interviews in particular may be a useful tool in the psychiatric examination of an individual, the courts have not generally recognized the trustworthiness and reliability of such tests as being sufficiently well-established to accord the results the status of competent evidence.[6]

Silving summarizes the legal criticism of these scientific tests as follows, "Recently, the proposition has been advanced that in exchange for apparently slight modification of established democratic processes of law, science will supply a method of highly reliable objective 'truth' finding by court experts."[7] She feels the fundamental question is the philosophical one involving our goal of attaining objective truth through the sacrifice of the dignity of the individual. She recalls the use of torture in previous

---

* Inbau has indicated that in lie detector tests the results are "indefinite" in 15 percent to 20 percent of the cases.[4]

days as the best means of proving guilt by confession and maintains,

> the danger of a similar development of objective testing, once its results are admitted, is very real. Public confidence in the omniscience of "science" is greater than the trust medieval man placed in torture as a method of eliciting truth. There can hardly be any doubt that as soon as expert testimony as to the results of psychological tests is, in principle, admitted, the weight of procedure will shift from the courtroom to the testing laboratory. The psychiatrist will became the real judge. Moreover, like torture, psychological testing cannot be conducted in public. Where the issues are decided in the laboratory, the institution of public trial is obviously a farce.[7]

Indeed, physicians themselves have struggled with the ethical and moral problems connected with their involvement in legal procedures. Macdonald asks, "Should a physician, on the request of police, administer drugs to a suspect for the purpose of obtaining a confession?"[8] The legal position in England is that a doctor shares with other citizens the duty to assist in the detection and arrest of a person who has committed a serious crime.

Guttmacher states the medical position as follows:

> An ethical and legal problem of increasing importance which concerns the clinical psychologist as well as the psychiatrist is the limits to which one may go in probing the unconscious of the defendant prior to trial by means of drugs, the so-called truth sera, hypnosis, lie detector and with the still more subtle device-projective clinical psychological techniques.[2]

Thus the legal and medical issues involved are complex and apparently disturbing; yet the need for continued and increasing use of psychiatric aids in the determination of truth has established their place in our judicial system. What is the current legal status of these tests for truth and what have psychiatrists and others been able to determine by their use?

When any of these tests for truth and validity of confession has been used in a criminal proceeding, the court generally has not allowed the results to be admitted in evidence. In an early case in California, the court refused to admit statements made by a defendant while hypnotized.[9] In another case, the defendant was interrogated while in an hypnotic trance by a psychologist in the presence of his defense attorney, concerning his implication in a murder. The court held that a recording made of such interrogation was not admissible in evidence, over objection of the prosecutor, pointing out that no case had been found permitting similar evidence to be introduced.[10]

Hypnosis has been employed to refresh memory, recall incidents, explore and explain motives, and determine truth or falsity; because the person hypnotized must submit voluntarily and be completely cooperative in order to make the medium successful, the question of duress or coercion is thereby eliminated. However, because of the required cooperation, some courts have disallowed hypnosis on the basis that it tends to be hearsay and self-serving evidence. This rationale has also been utilized in disallowing statements made under sodium amytal with prior consent.[11]

In recent cases, however, courts have allowed evidence based on narcoanalysis to be utilized in forming an opinion by the expert witness. In *People v. Jones* the court of appeals reversed exclusion of psychiatric testimony based on sodium pentothal tests by stating: "The proferred evidence was not the answers to certain questions but the interrogator's expert analysis of those answers for the purpose of determining whether (defendant) . . . was a sexual deviate."[12]

In *People v. Esposito* the opinion of the psychiatrist as to sanity or insanity of the defendants was admissible even though the opinion was based in part upon a sodium amytal interview. The court observed that it was not the admissibility of the defendant's statements or admissions, but the doctor's opinion which was involved; it found evidence in the record that psychiatrists regularly diagnosed mental illness by use of narcoanalysis.[13]

Although direct records from lie detector tests are not admissible as evidence in court, the polygraph machine has been used to obtain confessions in various ways. In *Commonwealth v. Hipple* a confession obtained employing a lie detector by police officers, otherwise voluntary, was admissible in evidence, since the record of the lie detector was not offered in evidence. The court said, "The statement by the officers, 'you can lie to us, but you cannot lie to this machine,' amounted to no more than an admonition to tell the truth," which was proper, and pointed out that, ". . . a confession procured by trick or artifice not calculated to produce an untruth, is never vitiated thereby."[14]*

In summary then, the psychiatric tests used in the search for truth must meet the following legal standards.

  a. They must be taken voluntarily and with proper consent by the accused to ensure protection under the constitutional right of due process of law.
  b. They must be used only as an adjunct to complete psychiatric evaluation; direct words obtained during the testing must never be offered in evidence in order to protect the accused from self-incrimination under the safeguards of the Fifth Amendment.
  c. They must never be utilized for the purpose of proving the truth of the matter or the guilt or innocence of the accused, as this use would usurp the function and duty of the jury.

Thus, even with the help of scientific aids, truth, in our judicial system, must be approached indirectly and tangentially as a part of expert medical opinion. How do these judicial demands and restrictions with regard to psychiatric tests correlate with recent medical findings?

First of all, the effect of drugs such as scopolamine, sodium pentothal and sodium amytal, generally, is to diminish the fear and anxiety of the patient by depression of his perceptive and integrative functions. This tends to produce a more relaxed state of mind and to permit the patient to talk more freely. In addition, the drugs facilitate temporary regression to less mature levels of personality integration and identification with the interrogator.[15]

Ludwig reported a study of malingering soldiers in whom he

---

* See M. Koessler, "The Admissibility of Confessions Obtained by Trickery," Am Bar Ass'n J, 50:648 (July, 1964). "Basing a conviction on a confession obtained by deceit is not only questionable as a matter of due process of law, but also involves the danger that the confession may be untrue and thus be the source of a miscarriage of justice."

found a persistence of negativistic attitudes and lack of communication even under narcosis.[16] A later study by Gerson and Victoroff analyed confessions obtained during narcoanalysis in which they found that fantasies and delusions which frequently could not be distinguished from reality significantly limited the credibility of statements.[17]

The study conducted at Yale by Redlich and others revealed the following conclusions with regard to the use of narcoanalysis: (a) "normal" patients under the influence of sodium amytal are not very likely to confess to wrong behavior; (b) neurotics are not only likely to confess to wrong behavior, but even tend to substitute fantasy for truth; (c) persons with strong unconscious self-punitive tendencies, such as moral masochists, not only confess more easily but also confess to crimes never actually committed; (d) narcoanalysis is occasionally effective in persons who would have disclosed the truth even without narcoanalysis. Conversely, suspects who would not ordinarily confess under skillful interrogation without drugs are just as likely to continue the deception while under the influence of drugs.[15]

Experimental and clinical findings indicate that only individuals who have conscious and unconscious reasons for doing so are inclined to confess and yield to interrogation under drug influence. Some are able to withhold information and some, especially character neurotics, are able to lie. Drugs are not "truth sera." They lessen inhibition to verbalization and stimulate unrepressed expression not only of fact, but fancy and suggestion as well. Thus, the material is not "truth" in the sense that it conforms to the empirical fact.[17]

All authorities are convinced that narcoanalysis is extremely helpful to the psychiatrist who may analyze the result of the narcoanalytic interview along with other scientific tests and observations which may provide him with a basis for psychiatric evaluation and therapy.

Narcoanalysis, when correctly used, may enable psychiatrists to probe more deeply and quickly in the psychological character of the subject. The results should not be regarded as "truth" but simply as clinical data "to be integrated with and interpreted in light of what is known concerning the dynamics of the subject's conflictual anxieties, motivation and behavioral tendencies."[15]

With regard to polygraph tests, Inbau feels there is only 5 percent error with skillful interpretation of data and Arthur has reported even less in his five year study.[4] Others, however, point out that the polygraph is not a lie detector *per se* and that there are many problems involved in the practical application of the polygraph techniques to the detection of deception.

> In crime detection the usual and obvious assumption of the investigator is that the subject either did or did not commit the alleged act and that deviations in the autonomic responses reflect conscious deviation in his verbal statements from the "truth" as the "truth" is conceived by the examiner. Laboratory and field studies have shown that this assumption is not always valid. There are many variables other than "intent to deceive" that can produce the observed results.[18]

The concept of "truth" is not easily defined; nor is the concept of "lying" any easier to classify. Perhaps "truth" ought to be considered in relative terms.

Guttmacher summarizes well the medical position. "Admittedly, the dividing line between truth and untruth is a shadowy one. It is debatable whether psychology and psychiatry have progressed to the point where they are able (with or without narcoanalysis) to establish the truth or falsity of testimony."[2]

Basically, then, medical evidence agrees with the caution expressed by the courts in limiting the use of psychiatric tests and techniques in the search for truth. The polygraph machine is not really a "lie detector," sodium amytal and sodium pentothal are not really "truth sera," and psychiatrists and psychologists are not "mind readers." However, appropriate use of these techniques by skilled clinicians can be quite helpful to the law in the evaluation of an individual and his behavior. Further implications of psychiatric intervention beyond this goal involve philosophical and political issues, a full discussion of which is beyond the scope of this treatise.

For example, the concept of free will and its limitation by use of drugs influencing confessions has been raised by many. One response to this criticism was expressed by Bauer, who maintains that the application of drugs to an examinee does not deprive him of his freedom of will, but by bringing his repressed material to consciousness, he is made truly free.[5]

Most psychiatrists avoid this free will determinance argument and do not speak of free will but rather degrees of freedom depending on the severity of neurosis; i.e. freedom to realize capabilities that were blocked by neurotic affliction. Freedom to choose is enhanced as one becomes unfettered of his neurotic bonds.

However, the question is raised, even where completely voluntary, is it proper for an individual to freely will to abandon his free will under the influence of drugs? Most authors have agreed with Frankfurter, who feels any deprivation of freedom of consent is not in keeping with our principles of justice and law. "The question (is) whether the behavior of the state's law enforcement officials was such as to overbear petitioner's will to resist and bring about confessions not fully self-determined, a question to be answered with complete disregard of whether or not petitioner in fact spoke the truth."[19]

A social/political/philosophical approach is expressed by Despres. "The involuntary use of such drugs on criminal suspects is premature until society fully accepts the principle and practice that law-breakers are to be treated and corrected, rather than punished, and that the aim of criminal administration should be the speedy cure, rehabilitation and restoration of the criminal without regard to traditional ideas of retribution and public punishment."[20]

Thus, psychiatrists have a difficult task to continue paving the road to their involvement in legal decisions, and in aiding the law in the determination of truth. There is a place for psychiatric and scientific aids in the law, but this place is and must be limited to the clinical evaluation of an individual as a patient with all due consideration of medical duty and public responsibility.

REFERENCES

1. Polen, E.: The admissibility of truth serum tests in the courts. *Temple Law Q*, 35:401, 1962.

2. Guttmacher, M.: *The Mind of the Murderer*. New York, Grove Press, 1962.
3. Szasz, T.: Mind-tapping: Psychiatric subversion of constitutional rights. *Am J Psychiat, 119*:323, Oct., 1962.
4. Inbau, F.: *Lie Detection and Criminal Interrogation*. Baltimore, Williams & Wilkins, 1942.
5. *State v. Lowry*, 163, Kan. 622, 185 P 2d 147 (1947).
6. *Henderson v. The State*, 94, Okla. Crim. 230 P 2d, 485, 502 (1951).
7. Silving, H.: Testing of the unconscious in criminal cases. *Harv L Rev, 69*:683, 1955.
8. MacDonald, J. M.: The use of drugs in the examination of suspected criminals. *J of Forensic Med, 3*:2, 1956.
9. *People v. Ebanks*, 117, Cal. 632, 49 P. 1049, 40 LRA 269.
10. *State v. Pusch*, 47, NW 2d 508 (N.D. 1950).
11. *People v. McNichol*, 100 Cal. App. 2d 554, 224, P. 2d 21.
12. *People v. Jones*, 42, Cal. 2d, 219, 266, P. 2d 38.
13. *People v. Esposito*, 287, NY 389, 39, NE 2d 925, 142 ALR 946 (1942).
14. *Comm. v. Hipple*, 333, Pa. 33, 3A 353 (1939).
15. Redlich, F. C., Ravitz, L. J., and Dession, G. H.: Narcoanalysis and truth. *Am J Psychiat, 107*:586, 1950.
16. Ludwig, A. O.: Clinical features and diagnosis of malingering in military personnel. *War Medicine, 5*:378, 1944.
17. Gerson, M. J., and Victoroff, V. M.: Experimental investigation into the validity of confession obtained under Sodium Amytal narcosis. *Clin Psychopathology, 9*:359, 1948.
18. Dearman, H. B., and Smith, B. M.: Unconscious motivation and the polygraph test. *Am J Psychiat, 119*:1017, May, 1963.
19. *Rogers v. Richmond*, 365, US 534, 540 (1961).
20. Despres, L. M.: Legal aspects of drug-induced statements. *U Chi L Rev, 14*:601, 616, 1947.

Section II
THE PSYCHIATRIST AND CRIMINAL LAW

THIS SECTION IS COMPRISED of seven chapters, four of which have been previously published in professional journals. In this section I have attempted to guide the attorney and the psychiatrist through the stages of criminal procedure and to highlight some of the difficulties that psychiatrists have in working in the criminal legal system. I have not delved into the philosophy or problems involved in tests of criminal responsibility or engaged in the usual debate regarding psychiatry's role in the courtroom. Rather, I have tried to bring to the practicing attorney and the interested psychiatrist some of the specific criminal problems they may face in working with individuals who have become involved in criminal proceedings. This section is a practical one; it does not deal in the philosophy or academics of the psychiatric role in the criminal process.

Chapter 7

MENTAL ILLNESS AND THE CRIMINAL PROCESS: ROLE OF THE PSYCHIATRIST

RECENT DECISIONS by the United States Supreme Court[1] increasingly have indicated the need for adequate legal counsel in early stages of the criminal process to the point where one may ask, "Ought the arresting police officer be more completely trained in the law?" Or, "Ought society provide a lawyer in every police car to be available at the time of arrest?" Indeed, how early in the criminal procedure must the suspect or defendant have legal counsel? The same question also is becoming more significant with respect to the role of the psychiatrist in the criminal procedure; i.e. at what stages is the determination of mental illness by expert opinion a significant feature in the criminal process?

Traditionally, the psychiatrist was called upon to evaluate suspects or defendants with respect to the following.

    a. determination of present insanity based on mental illness; i.e. whether the defendant is able to understand the nature of the charges against him and able to cooperate in his own defense.

    b. determination of criminal responsibility at the time of the offense; i.e. evaluation of mental status at an earlier time to ascertain whether the defendant was suffering from mental disease or defect such that he did not know the nature and quality of the act he is alleged to have done and did not know that what he was doing was wrong.[2]

    c. recommendation for disposition by the court after findings;

Originally published in the *American Bar Association Journal*, 54:566, June, 1968.

i.e. the determination that defendant, though not insane according to the legal tests employed at trial, is suffering from mental disease or disorder such that incarceration in a prison would aggravate his condition, or that he is in need of treatment in a mental hospital.

d. recommendation for stay of execution of sentence, especially with respect to capital punishment; i.e. the medical finding that the individual is suffering from mental illness such that he does not know why he is being executed.*

These four stages in criminal procedure are certainly the crucial ones in which the determination of mental status plays a most significant role. However, it is submitted that there are other stages in the entire gamut of the criminal process where psychiatric evaluation and consultation is highly significant. The purpose of this chapter is to discuss these stages in which the evaluation of mental status is warranted and in which the service of a psychiatrist is indicated.

The Criminal Offense

The criminal act itself forms the initial stage of the criminal procedure, for without the act, there is no crime; but without criminal intent, also there is no crime, for the crime consists of the *actus reus* and the *mens rea*. Thus, determination of mental capacity to form the evil intent is material to every crime, though in practice it is often overlooked or is assumed to be present.

Evaluation of the offender's mental status at the time of commission of his criminal act usually is unavailable directly and must be determined at some later time after arrest. The offender is assumed by law to possess normal mental capacity to form a *mens rea* or guilty intent unless proven otherwise by expert testimony. The offender may be shown to have sufficient mental disease at the time of the offense such that he did not meet the legal criteria of the appropriate test for criminal responsibility

---

* The rationale is humanistic but also the historical notion exists that if the convicted and about-to-be sentenced individual were mentally well, he might be able to provide a last minute clue to his innocence.

for the jurisdiction in which the offense was committed. In crimes requiring specific intent, such as burglary, the ability to form such intent is assumed, unless the defendant is found to be suffering from disease of the mind (regardless of cause) preventing the formation of such specific intent.[3]

In most instances a formal presentation of the medical findings of mental status at time of the initial stage of the criminal process must await the later judicial stage in which they are utilized in the exculpatory plea.

The Investigatory Phase

Determination of mental status by the psychiatrist seems of special significance in two problems that might be encountered in the investigation phase of criminal process.

First, the consent to search and seizure without a warrant by a suspect may be vitiated by evidence of mental incompetency to give such consent. This may be an issue when the suspect is obviously mentally ill, but is more important when he is mentally ill such that only an experienced psychiatrist can tell with any degree of certainty.*

Perhaps of greater concern in the investigatory phase involves obtaining confessions from suspects who are mentally ill.

> In the case at bar, the evidence indisputably establishes the strongest probability that Blackburn was insane and incompetent at the time he allegedly confessed. Surely in the present stage of our civilization a most basic sense of justice is affronted by the spectacle of incarcerating a human being upon the basis of a statement he made while insane; a misjudgment can without difficulty be articulated in terms of the unreliability of the confession, the lack of rational choice of the accused, or simply a strong conviction that our system

---

* A similar problem occurred in 1957 when a state police officer drew a blood sample from the defendant while he was unconscious. The analysis of the sample was admitted into evidence in a state prosecution for manslaughter. See *Breithaupt v. Abram,* 352, U.S. 432 (1957). Two state courts have held that such taking of blood is an unreasonable search and siezure under the Fourth Amendment. See *State v. Wolf* (Del) 164, A 2d 865 (1960) and *State v. Kroenig* (Wisc) 79, NW 2d, 810 (1957). Query: Is it also an unreasonable "search and seizure" if the defendant was not unconscious but mentally incompetent to give proper consent?

of law enforcement should not operate so as to take advantage of a person in this fashion.[4]

Voluntary confessions by mentally incompetent persons, when the officer is not trying to obtain a confession, but is only making inquiries, poses a difficult problem, especially in heinous crimes that are well publicized.†

The Accusatory Phase

The accusatory phase includes the arrest with further investigation, the preliminary arraignment, the preliminary hearing and the indictment by the grand jury. The problem of confession is even more significant in the early accusatory phase when the defendant is incarcerated and interrogated. The use of various devices for obtaining confessions for arriving at the "truth," such as lie detector tests, truth sera and psychiatric interviews with psychological testing, is of crucial importance. It should be stressed that none of these devices has been shown to produce the "truth" and the results of their use cannot be relied upon in a judicial proceeding.[5]

Furthermore, their use may present a danger to the suspect or defendant and must be supervised by competent professionals. Certainly the use of any "truth detecting" devices in insane or incompetent individuals is to be prohibited. An example of the misuse of a psychiatrist in this phase of investigation is well exhibited by the case of *People v. Leyra,* where a psychiatrist posed as a friend or helping individual to seduce the defendant to confess. This method of obtaining confession was found to be in violation of the individual's rights by the Supreme Court of the United States after the confession was originally admitted in evidence.[6]

The right to counsel usually begins after the arrest and during investigation, prior to confession. The consent to waiver of right to counsel at this stage or waiver of this legal right may be vitiated by determination of mental incompetency to so waive

---

† Mostly, these people who confess to "popular crimes" are guilt-ridden individuals looking for punishment and are only too eager to "admit" they "must be responsible" for the crime and request to be imprisoned.

at this point. It is submitted that proper psychiatric evaluation of defendants at this stage in the legal process presents a greater opportunity for appropriate administration of justice rather than waiting for the preliminary judicial phase, as is traditionally done.

As soon as the defense counsel becomes involved in the proceedings, the psychiatrist may be called in appropriate cases to evaluate the defendant. In private cases this is usually no problem as counsel is called at time of arrest and the examining doctor is well compensated for his time and services. However, in the case of indigent defendants, the voluntary defender may or may not be present at the preliminary hearing. Indeed, according to Goldstein:

> In most jurisdictions no provision is made for appointment of counsel at this stage. Neither the due process clause of the Fourteenth Amendment nor state constitutional provisions have been held to require this. And most states make no statutory provision for appointment of counsel, though a considerable number require that he be advised of his right to retain counsel. Since, therefore, defense counsel is usually either not present or not sufficiently informed to play his role properly, it ordinarily falls to the magistrate, almost alone, to test the sufficiency of the evidence to warrant holding the accused for the grand jury, or for trial, where there is no grand jury. Yet most magistrates are either unskilled or too busy, or too closely linked with police or prosecutor, to be sufficiently mindful of the "judicial" nature of their role to perform this function adequately. And the sole review of the sufficiency of the evidence before them is the limited one afforded by *habeas corpus,* which looks only for some "legally competent evidence" to support the order committing the accused for trial. But even that is a limited safeguard because the unrepresented, or poorly represented, defendant, may not learn until after his trial that there was insufficient evidence at the preliminary hearing to warrant passing the case on to trial. If the case has proceeded to trial, no remedy is available to the accused for the defect in the preliminary hearing. He must then look on appeal solely to the inadequacy of the evidence at trial.[7]

Thus, the defendant deprived of counsel is also deprived of the availability of adequate psychiatric examination, the results of which could be sufficient to mitigate or vitiate the "probable cause" necessary at this early stage of the criminal process.

What is needed, then, is the official machinery to authorize counsel for indigent defendants at the preliminary hearing. Even if counsel could be provided at this stage, though, does he have access to psychiatric opinion? The answer is almost invariably no. The court psychiatric clinics are not geared for this early evaluation. Even if the psychiatrists in the court clinic could be available for evaluation during the preliminary hearing, their reports would not be the closed, confidential consultations that are available in similar private cases. Thus, what is needed is a community psychiatric resource from which voluntary defender may draw for such evaluation and consultation; preferably he should have on his staff a psychiatrist who would be in a position to render this valuable service.*

The significance of early psychiatric evaluation lies in several areas. First, probable cause may be vitiated by insanity. Second, proper commitment procedures may be instituted at the early phase, thus eliminating the expensive judicial proceedings and clearing the court calendar for other criminal cases. Third, preventing the stigma of indictment and the stress of adjudication plus instituting proper psychiatric help at the earliest time may be invaluable aids to proper and rapid recovery. Prognosis for recovery in many cases is improved by early treatment and elimination of undue stress and strain. Finally, the decision whether or not to prosecute is that of the district attorney, based on his opinion of the evidence at hand. It is suggested that psychiatric opinion at this stage would provide the district attorney with further significant evidence on which to base his decision.

Thus early psychiatric involvement is appropriate and helpful to both the individual accused and to society and should become available where indicated. The administrative disposition of appropriate cases at this stage of preliminary examination would

---

* The Unit in Law and Psychiatry at Temple University had established a Forensic Psychiatry Clinic for such purposes. During the first five months of operation, forty-three individuals were referred by the Defender Association, of whom forty were evaluated and consultation provided. Eighteen of the forty (45%) were referred for pretrial evaluation; none was requested at the early preliminary hearings, because most defendants were not represented by defense counsel until after arraignment and/or indictment.

save time and expense that is currently being utilized in the later judicial phases of the criminal procedure.

The Preliminary Judicial Phase

This phase includes the post-indictment period and the arraignment with defendant's plea. This is the stage in the criminal process in which psychiatrists traditionally have been called to evaluate the defendants, with respect to present insanity and criminal responsibility.

Historically, the first advisory court clinic was inaugurated by Dr. William Healy in the Cook County Juvenile Court of Chicago in 1909. In 1914 the first adult court psychiatric clinic was established in Chicago and in 1921 the first compulsory, court-affiliated psychiatric service was established in Massachusetts under the "Briggs Law" which provided that an individual accused of certain offenses must be given a psychiatric examination within forty-eight hours after indictment by a court-appointed psychiatrist. It was applicable in capital offenses and in cases where a person had been indicted more than once for any other offense, or had been previously convicted of a felony.[8]

During this phase the question of competency to stand trial arises with its criteria of ability to understand the nature of the charges against the defendant and the ability to cooperate in his own defense; i.e. "mental competency" or "present insanity." This determination is a much more appropriate task for the psychiatrist than the question of responsibility, since the evaluation of mental status forms a part of every "routine" psychiatric examination. The difference is the translation of medical findings to the legal questions posed above, thus becoming a matter of psychiatric judgment and opinion.

In practice, psychiatrists rarely disagree about present insanity or mental incompetency to stand trial, and if the psychiatrist called by defense counsel is prepared to testify that the defendant is incompetent to stand trial, his statements usually are not challenged by the district attorney and an agreement is made for civil commitment, at the termination of which the trial may be held.

This kind of administrative cooperation and disposition that benefits both society and the individual should serve as a model for further use in less clear-cut situations; e.g. in questions of mental illness, short of incompetency, short of insanity, but nevertheless of significant severity to have contributed greatly to criminal offensive behavior. As discussed in the earlier phase, must we impose a verdict of guilty on these individuals to make their tenuous adjustment even more difficult? An administrative decision in cooperation with judge, defense counsel and prosecuting attorney with reference to disposition without verdict in many cases would prove more feasible both to society and to the defendant.

Dr. Bernard Diamond, a noted forensic psychiatrist, presents this position in terms of "diminished responsibility" in criminal behavior.

> The next step is to expand the principle of limited or diminished responsibility of the mentally ill offender to include definitions of crime. It was easier to introduce this principle in the crimes of homicide because there already exists in the legal structure a graduated responsibility for homicide, but when the courts, and particularly the public, get used to the idea of giving full consideration to the mental and emotional abnormalities of the homicide offender, there will be little difficulty in having the same principles and practices applied to all crimes. We would then have diminished responsibility in its true meaning, extending throughout the penal code and no longer bound to the technicalities of the degree of homicide.[9]

The Later Judicial Phase

This phase of the criminal process includes the trial with exculpatory plea, plea in bar of sentence and presentence investigation following guilty verdict.

Again, traditionally, psychiatrists have been called upon to provide expert testimony with respect to the defendant's degree of mental responsibility at the time of the offense. This may be a difficult task and must be done indirectly at some time after the offense. At best, the psychiatrist can only assume within the limits of his expertise, what the mental status was at that earlier time, but can never be absolutely certain since he did not examine the defendant at that time. This determination has proved troublesome both for psychiatrists and lawyers as well as for judges and juries. Much has been written on the difficulties involved and the "impossible" position in which the psychiatrist often is placed.

Diamond again reflects the difficulty of the psychiatric position.

> Whenever a psychiatrist is called upon to testify, under the M'Naghten Rule of knowledge of right and wrong, as to the sanity or insanity of a defendant, the psychiatrist must either renounce his own values with all their medical-humanistic application and thereby becoming a puppet doctor, used by the law to further the punitive and vengeful goals demanded by our society; or he must commit perjury if he accepts the literal definition of the M'Naghten Rule. If he tells the truth—stating on the witness stand that just about every defendant, no matter how mentally ill, no matter how advanced his psychosis, knows the difference between right and wrong, in the literal sense of the phrase—he becomes an expeditor to the gallows or gas chamber.[9]

Recently, various jurisdictions have modified the requirements of the rules for expert psychiatric testimony. Many have provided for full psychiatric testimony, a situation which has obtained in the military proceedings for some time.

Historically, since 1926 California has utilized "split trial" when questions of insanity arose. Under this procedure, the defendant is conclusively presumed sane for the purpose of the first trial. If he is found "guilty" at that trial, then a second trial is held to determine if he is sane or insane.*

The rationale for adopting the split trial was expressed by the 1925 Commission for the Reform of Criminal Procedure.

> The abuses of the present system are great. Under a plea of "not guilty" and without any notice to the people that the defense of insanity will be relied upon, defendant has been able to raise the defense upon the trial of the issue as to whether he committed the offense charged. This lack of notice that such a defense would be made has very frequently placed the people at a very great disadvantage. An even more serious fault of the present system is that a defendant when on trial as to whether he committed the offense, is

---

* California Penal Code, §1026.

able to bring into the case the whole matter of insanity at the time of the offense charged. This enables him to submit to the jury great masses of evidence having no bearing upon the question whether the offense was committed. This frequently is made the basis of appeals to the sympathy or prejudice of the jury and even though this is not done, often introduces a great confusion into the trial.[10]

However, a more recent commission in California studying the problem states, "We have serious doubts whether these reasons were sound in 1927; in any event we think they are unsound today . . . in short, the split trial is no longer serving a useful purpose; we think it should be abandoned."[10]

With respect to current changes in the rules providing for psychiatric testimony, Diamond states,

The effect will be, I am certain, to encourage the psychiatrist to practice as good medicine in the courtroom as he does in his own office and hospital. In essence the court will say to the expert witness: "Forget about the legal definitions and the technicalities, forget about sanity or insanity; premeditation, malice and *mens rea*—that is our concern. Tell us everything you as a medical expert know about this defendant. What kind of person is he? What is wrong with him emotionally and mentally? How did he get to be the way he is now? What made him do what he is accused of? What hidden mechanisms in his mind caused him to behave the way he did? What kind of treatment does he need to ensure his rehabilitation? Is he likely to respond to treatment? What kind of protection does society require to prevent something like this happening again? Tell us all that you know about the defendant and we will give full consideration to what you have said; we will put it together with all of the evidence from other sources; then we will decide what is best for society to do with this defendant."[9]

Perhaps one of the most significant innovations of this phase of the criminal process has been the broadened use of presentence investigations, utilizing psychiatric and other investigators. The psychiatrist serves as the head of a team of clinical investigators collecting social, family, vocational, psychological and psychiatric data that are presented to the court as a significant aid in making a proper disposition. This service is the traditional one provided by the court psychiatric clinic. The late Dr. Manfred Guttmacher, formerly Medical Director of the Clinic of the Court of Baltimore, pointed out, "Half of the criminal cases referred to the Baltimore Court Clinic have already been found guilty. The Clinic's task in these cases is to advise the court in regard to disposition and sentence. We believe that psychiatry can make its greatest contribution to criminal justice at this point."[11]

There is no question that this forensic service is the one for which the psychiatrist is most fully trained by traditional methods and in which he feels most competent and least threatened. A relatively recent addition to the advisory service regarding disposition of offenders has occurred with the passing, since 1937 in two thirds of the states, the so-called "Sexual Psychopath Statutes." Under provision of these statutes, the recidivistic sexual offender who presents a menace to society may be sentenced to an indeterminate period ranging from one day to life.

This provision raises the question of dangerousness of the offender and the proper disposition of the "dangerous offender" for the protection of society. The determination has been elusive and presents a significant area of research for the continued cooperative efforts of psychiatry and the law.*

The Post-Sentence Phase

The post-sentence phase, still a part of the judicial phase, since the trial judge maintains jurisdiction over the inmate, is an often forgotten stage of criminal procedure. This phase includes incarceration and parole, both of which lend well to psychiatric involvement.

The role of the psychiatrist in correctional institutions has become increasingly important and significant. Psychiatric treatment of offenders is part of the total rehabilitation program as an accepted feature of corrections. In addition, psychiatrists are asked to evaluate inmates with respect to recommendations for transfer, parole, commitment to mental institutions, types of vocational possibilities, further extramural psychotherapy and the traditional evaluation of mental competency for execution of capital punishment.

---

* For a more complete discussion of "dangerousness" see Chapter 9.

Psychiatric consultation to the parole board in cases where parolees are having a difficult adjustment based on emotional disturbances has proven to be of value though it is not available in most areas. Furthermore, treatment of parolees, by group therapy and individual therapy, with medication when appropriate, has been extremely helpful in keeping these men on parole and out of prison. Specifically, it is helpful if the psychiatrist who treats the inmate in the correctional institution is available to follow-up with extramural treatment when on parole. The continuity of this relationship is of benefit to a more stable extramural adjustment.

Summary and Conclusions

The role of the psychiatrist in the criminal process traditionally has been in the middle phases. Too little psychiatric intervention at the early stages of the proceedings is apparent. It is suggested that this situation be remedied by providing for psychiatric evaluation at the preliminary hearing, when appropriate. In addition, the psychiatrist has not been as involved in the later rehabilitative stages, as he might well be. It is felt that the psychiatrist can make a significant contribution during these later phases by providing evaluation to the parole board and treatment to the parolees and probationers.

The traditional functions of the psychiatrist in the criminal process can be intensified and improved upon as well as expanded to include the earliest and latest phases. Generally, the psychiatrist should be available for consultation in all phases of the criminal process.

REFERENCES

1. *Gideon v. Wainwright*, 372, U.S. 335 (1963) and *Escobedo v. Illinois*, 378, U.S. 478 (1964).
2. M'Naghten's Case, 10 Clark and Finney, 2008 *Eng Rep* 718 (1843).
3. *Fisher v. U.S.*, 328 U.S. 463 (1946).
4. *Blackburn v. U.S.*, 361, U.S. 199, 206-7 (1959).
5. Sadoff, R. L.: Psychiatric involvement in the search for truth. *Am Bar Assoc J*, 52:251-4, March, 1966.
6. *New York v. Leyra*, 302 NY 353 98 NE 2d 553 (1951). *Leyra v. Denno*, 347, US 556 (1954). *New York v. Leyra*, 1, NY 2d 199, 134, NE 2d 475 (1956).

7. Goldstein, A. S.: The state of the accused: Balance of advantage in criminal procedure. *Yale Law J*, 69:1149, 1156, 1960.
8. Massachusetts Law, TER, Ed. C 123, 100A (1932).
9. Diamond, B. L.: Criminal responsibility and the mentally ill. *Stanford L Rev, 14*:59, Dec., 1961.
10. Special Commission on Insanity and Criminal Offenders, State of California, First Report, July 7, 1962.
11. Guttmacher, M. S., and Weihofen, H.: *Psychiatry and the Law.* New York, Norton, 1952.

Chapter 8

CRIMINAL BEHAVIOR MASKING MENTAL ILLNESS

THE RELATIONSHIP BETWEEN mental illness and criminal behavior is a complex one; numerous attempts have been made to classify and integrate criminal behavior into accepted psychosocial diagnoses. On the one extreme, some psychiatrists consider all criminals to be mentally disturbed; on the other, crime is viewed primarily as a social illness. In between, various combinations and associations have been put forth. This chapter will present brief summaries of five cases of individuals committing various crimes who utilized the criminal-legal structure and process as a means of attempted resolution of emotional conflicts. None may be considered a "professional criminal type," and most intended to obscure their mental disturbance by criminal behavior. One found it necessary to engage in criminal acts in order to call attention to his illness.

CASE PRESENTATIONS

Case Number One

Bob is a twenty-one-year-old single, Mexican-American Indian, private in the U.S. Army, stationed in Germany. He was charged with homicide and aggravated assault with intent to kill, during a knife fight outside a taproom in Germany. He had been drinking fairly heavily and did not know exactly what had occurred, but came away from the area with a knife which he believed to be responsible for the homicide. He hid the knife in the ground near his bunk, but did not think he had stabbed anyone. He did not wish to get anyone into trouble.

Reprinted with permission from *Corrective Psychiatry & Journal of Social Therapy*, 17:41, No. 2, 1971.

Criminal Behavior Masking Mental Illness

During the preliminary investigation of the homicide, Bob denied his involvement and did not reveal the location of the knife. During the next several months he began to use psychedelic drugs, and hashish, which he had used even prior to the fight. Also prior to the fight he had taken one dose of LSD and experienced a "bad trip," including hallucinations, without taking any further doses of LSD.

About six months after the killing, Bob began to note that people were demanding things of him and yelling at him at various times. He was afraid he was going crazy, but chose to deny it and tried to ignore the symptoms. The hallucinations became more pronounced; there were many times when he was unable to sleep properly and seemed to look unusual or weird to his friends. He described such episodes as falling out in formation when no one else was present, and imagining that his sergeant was giving him orders to drill, which he would do alone.

He confessed that he was aware of his emotional and mental difficulties but was afraid to see a doctor for fear he would be placed in a hospital. He had a profound fear of psychiatrists and mental hospitals since his aunt had become psychotic on the Indian Reservation in New Mexico where he was raised, and she was treated there by the "witch doctors."

At the time of the height of his psychosis he was scheduled to report to the Central Intelligence Division (CID) to identify others present at the fight six months previously. He experienced further hallucinations and panic on the bus trip to the CID office. He hallucinated that people were yelling at him and making further demands on him, and he wished only to get away from them. In his mind he felt the only way to get away was to be sent to the stockade and be locked up. He knew the only way to be locked up was to confess to the killing. His paranoia became flagrant to the point that he felt he could read other people's minds.

He felt in his psychotic state of mind that if he spent ten to fifteen years in jail his illness would leave him, he would be himself again and not subject to the same misery and hallucinations that he experienced prior to his arrest. He was arrested primarily on the basis of his confession with no external evidence; in fact, to the contrary, most witnesses testified that he was not involved in the fight and did not do the stabbing.

Psychiatric examination one year after the crime found him to be suffering from schizophrenic reaction, paranoid type, in partial remission. He had recovered sufficiently to tell the examiner about his fears of being diagnosed as psychotic. Bob chose consciously to be labeled as a criminal rather than a mentally ill person. He feared the label of psychosis because of his previous experiences with the type of treatment that he expected to receive. He felt it would be to his advantage to be locked up in prison for several years so that his illness would go away. At the time of his confession he was so disturbed that all he could think about was relief from his misery.

In Bob's case we see a flight into criminal confession as a means of avoiding treatment for serious psychotic mental illness. He was still convinced at the time of the interview that the only treatment for him was to spend long years in prison and that medicine and psychiatric treatment could not help his illness or his hallucinations. He felt if he were to leave the stockade he would undoubtedly be revisited with the hallucinations that caused him so much emotional distress and panic.

He was acquitted of all charges on the basis of the psychiatric evaluation and report providing a reasonable understanding of his mental condition to the court.

Case Number Two

Jim is a twenty-two-year-old single, white private in the U.S. Army, from a fairly well-to-do middle-class family, who had deserted to Sweden. His history is fairly unremarkable until the time he entered the military and had a complicated situation in Germany. He had used marijuana while on active duty without ill effect. He had manipulated the situation such that he was able to attend various schools and have special privileges within his unit. Because of the changes in the unit he began to feel persecuted and deprived of his special privileges. He blamed a jealous lieutenant whom he thought was interested in his girl friend. He felt he was taken advantage of on several occasions and improperly talked into reenlisting because he did not get the assignment that was promised. He also became involved in a homosexual relationship with two other men.

Although he said he had tried to make a "go of it" in the Army despite his feelings of persecution and unfairness, one day, under extreme pressure, he "walked away from the unit." He took a train to Frankfurt and flew to Sweden. In Sweden he was unable to find work, but met a girl whom he married and said he found "peace and harmony." His father and attorney both flew to Sweden to return him to the States to clear up his legal difficulties. He was forced to leave his wife in Sweden and promised faithfully to return to her. His existence he felt was incomplete without his wife. He wrote many poems about her, some of which were quite incomprehensible and reflected his psychotic thought disorder.

On one occasion he went AWOL from the stockade at a U.S. Army post and joined with a radical action group with whom he identified. He also identified with the radical movement in the U.S. and his intelligence allowed him to work effectively for them. He adopted an identity within the hippie subculture. His major goal in life was to return to Sweden to his wife, to give up the American ideals and to join radical movements in Europe.

Psychiatric examination revealed that Jim suffered from active hallucinations, felt he was invisible at times and showed inappropriate feeling tone. He was suspicious, guarded, evasive and generally had inappropriate thought content with psychotic ideation. Jim represents an example of a young man suffering from an acute psychotic reaction, paranoid schiophrenic type, with hallucinations and delusions, who suffered homosexual panic while in Europe, causing him to flee to Sweden.

In Sweden he found a subculture with which he could identify and deny his psychotic ideation. As long as he clung to the hippie subculture with his radical ideations and psychedelic experiences he could avoid the consideration of his own mental illness. It was only when he was returned to the United States in order to clear up his charges that Jim's psychosis reappeared.

In this case we have an example of an individual who was able to deny his mental illness by identifying with a group of people who shared his concerns and accusations against the United States Government. As long as he clung to that identity his mental illness could be avoided and denied. This is not to imply that all individuals who identify with the hippie subculture are necessarily psychotic or mentally ill. The majority, are not; however, there are some who are able to "fit in" with this group and effectively mask the psychotic processes that become more obvious in an authoritarian structure. In Jim's case it was essential to make this distinction though he continued to deny his illness.

Case Number Three

John is a twenty-nine-year-old single, unemployed male who was arrested for bank robbery. Initially he claimed that he robbed the bank for "suicidal purposes" and later indicated that he did it as a "plea for help." John had been in treatment in one of the large hospitals in Philadelphia and had left treatment in order to travel. While away he experienced a recurrence of his depressive feelings, with suicidal ideation. He sought treatment in another city but therapy was denied him because of administrative difficulties. He decided to return to Philadelphia in a bitter, angry mood. He felt inadequate, worthless and depressed. Upon returning he went immediately to the hospital that had previously treated him but was refused further treatment until he could be reevaluated at some later time.

He became fearful of an impending breakdown and "decided" that the only way to get help would be through arrest. He drank several beers, walked into a bank and handed the teller a note stating, "Give me all your five's and ten's or I'll blow your head off." He took the money, walked calmly out of the door, went ten steps, stopped and waited to be arrested. He was very cooperative at his arrest, no weapon was found, and he readily gave back the money, stating, "It's about time you got here; please take me to the hospital."

He was diagnosed as a schizoid personality disorder, manifesting bizarre fantasies, inability to form close personal relationships, aloofness and alienation to others, with overwhelming fears, but was found to be not psychotic. The principal concern that led to his depression and subsequent erratic behavior and panic was his fear that he was a homosexual.

John represents the case of an individual who was aware of his impending breakdown and sought help which was denied him. His conscious means of achieving the aid that he could not get voluntarily was to be arrested, i.e. to consider a legal or criminal disposition rather than a medical one. Though John was not psychotic, he was seriously mentally disturbed and chose a desperate means of obtaining necessary help.

Case Number Four

Joseph is a thirty-two-year-old married, father of two children who has been a narcotics addict for many years. He had attempted to get help for his problem but had never been able to stay in a voluntary hospital. His compulsive need for drugs, including psychedelics, was overwhelming, causing him to leave the hospital treatment center prematurely. One morning he did not go to work since he had taken LSD and marijuana and was "high" on his "trip." He injected one dose of heroin in order to come off the "trip" but found that to be insufficient. In a desperate attempt to get money for more heroin, Joseph walked into a bank and asked for ten thousand dollars, in a nonthreatening manner. He became frightened, experienced panic and started to run. He was arrested almost immediately in a confused state of mind.

Joseph was not aware of the underlying cause of his addiction; i.e. depression. Traditional psychotherapy programs were not helpful to him, since he could not remain in a voluntary treatment setting. Unconsciously he sought effective help for his illness by using the criminal-legal machinery via his uncontrollable need for drugs. His plea for help perhaps is not as obvious as John's, and one could not speculate that consciously he wanted to be arrested. He later confessed that he was desperate and needed to be "forced into treatment" involuntarily, since he could not allow himself to stay in a voluntary treatment setting. He saw only the drug habit as a problem but not the more serious and crippling depression which he masked by the use of drugs.

Case Number Five

Dick is a twenty-six-year-old, extremely effeminate, woman's clothing designer, who was arrested for sending obscene letters through the mail. He admits that he had sent about two hundred letters to people that he did not know, using the same wording in each of the letters, over the past ten years, indicating that he and several other men would "spread-eagle" the victim and one of them would insert his "long penis" into the victim's rectum. He described this in sadistic sexual terms, using obscene terminology. He could not understand his need to write the letters and said he had written them in spurts for several weeks or months at a time when he felt like doing so. On closer examination it was revealed that Dick had been sexually assaulted when he was sixteen years old. His assault was accurately reproduced in detail in his letters, except that he became the aggressor and not the victim. This reaction is similar to that observed in youngsters playing the role of physician following minor surgery.

His letter writing was viewed as an aid in the internal resolution of his fantasy that he had been emasculated. His becoming the aggressor in a fantasied act toward the others allowed him to handle the anxiety that often became overwhelming.

Dick represents an individual in whom a less serious crime was found to be the method of avoiding or denying the internal psychological conflicts that engulfed him. He could handle in part his conflict by writing letters and avoid dealing with his own internal fears. Once he was arrested, however, the problem became clearer and he was able to face up to the trauma that he experienced and receive adequate treatment, following which the letter writing ceased.

DISCUSSION

These five cases exemplify the phenomenon in which people accused of committing crimes have used the criminal-legal process as an indirect mechanism for handling internal conflicts. All utilize the legal process in a therapeutic manner to avoid facing their real difficulties, and receive some form of relief from their anxieties. People may handle anxiety or conflicts in a number of ways: they may be aware of and feel anxiety, they may convert the anxiety of physical symptoms, they may repress anxiety, or they may "act it out" in aberrant behavior.

Many of the case histories presented reflect examples of the individual "acting out" his internal conflicts in such a manner as to deny their existence and focus only on antisocial or criminal behavior. In this way the individual may avoid recognizing that which he wishes to hide. In some cases our criminal structure allows for successful self-deception and the conflicts remain unresolved. Recidivistic criminal behavior may then result.

The individual who uses the criminal-legal structure in order to obtain necessary treatment either because he feels he has been denied treatment, or because he cannot accept voluntary therapy programs, poses an even greater challenge. Here, the patient recognizes his underlying emotional difficulties but may be so aggressive, hostile and dangerous that the typical psychiatric facility is unable or unwilling to treat him. In some cases this rejection may encourage the individual to react in a criminal manner in order to have court-mandated or enforced psychiatric treatment.

We must be aware of underlying psychodynamic mechanisms in criminal behavior in order to prescribe proper disposition. It is not sufficient to say a person is not motivated for treatment because he cannot work in a voluntary rehabilitation program. Many people feel it is shameful to admit they need help and would never ask for treatment. However, if psychotherapy were mandated by a judge, they would accept it, feeling they were "forced to go." Psychiatrists traditionally have felt that motivation is essential to success in psychotherapy. However, results of "enforced psychotherapy" programs for probationers have been gratifying.[1]

Three of the cases presented used drugs illegally. Mostly, marijuana is used infrequently by the curious and rebellious youngster, but more regularly and with other more dangerous drugs by a few, who have need to obscure underlying conflicts. For this reason all individuals arrested for drug abuse should have benefit of psychiatric examination.

Summary

Five cases are presented to highlight underlying psychodynamic factors involved in criminal behavior and encourage use of psychiatric consultation where indicated. Criminal behavior may serve to mask or obscure mental illness and the criminal-legal structure may be "used" for such purpose. It is imperative that we learn to recognize when this phenomenon occurs, that we may work cooperatively to provide proper disposition. In this way we may attack the underlying conflicts that give rise to further difficulties and subsequent criminal behavior.

REFERENCES

1. Peters, J. J., Pedigo, J. M., Steg, J., and McKenna, J. J.: Group psychotherapy of the sex offender. *Federal Probation,* September, 1968.

Chapter 9

THE PSYCHIATRIST AND DANGEROUSNESS: PREDICTING VIOLENT BEHAVIOR

DANGEROUSNESS IN AN INDIVIDUAL is a pivotal issue in both criminal and civil cases. Its detection or prediction remains a key question for disposition or commitment of offenders and mentally ill persons.

Can a psychiatrist predict when and if a person will become violent or dangerous to himself or others? This is a most difficult question and raises a number of problems. There are factors that can be utilized to predict future violent behavior. Psychiatry depends primarily on intrapsychic conflicts, past history and diagnosis in making such predictions, but additionally there are a number of other elements in a person's life that need to be evaluated in making such predictions.

The problem of prediction becomes one of an art as well as a science. In reviewing the history of those who attempted to make such predictions about other people's behavior, we may start with those who read the stars and turn to those who read bumps on the head, called phrenologists, to those who read palms and other physical criteria, none of which bore any respectable fruit.

If we discount the external characteristics such as the sly look, the balding head, the warty hands, the red face and the individuals who utilize dreams as predictors of the future, we may turn to the group called "behaviorists" who would be able to predict future behavior on the basis of past actions, performances and behavior. This is primarily what criminologists and statisticians do; i.e. they utilize tables of prediction based on past performance and indicate that a burglar will have a great likelihood for recidivism, whereas homicide within a family has a low recidivism rate.

The Gluecks[1,2] many years ago had attempted to predict delinquency among a series of children they studied and followed for over ten years. Their predictions were quite accurate, based on their observations.

If we turn next to the dynamicists; i.e. the people who look to psychodynamics in the cause of certain types of behavior, we come to the modern day forensic psychiatric approach to criminality and the attendant issue of prediction of violent behavior.

A small book, edited by Dr. Jonas Rappeport,[3] entitled *The Clinical Evaluation of the Dangerousness of the Mentally Ill*, is a collection of papers presented at a symposium held several years ago. The group concluded that history of prior mental illness with hospitalization does not result in higher incidences of violent behavior. More recently, Dr. Melvin Heller of Temple University presented a paper at the first annual meeting (1969) of the American Academy of Psychiatry and the Law on the diagnosis of dangerousness. In his presentation, Dr. Heller alludes to the deceptiveness and duplicity of humans, with respect to their fellow man. He feels this type of treachery is an important element in the survival of the human species with respect to other animals. He considers that man basically is potentially dangerous but that there are special circumstances under which one is more likely to act violently. He says we should consider a wide variety of criteria, including past history, current life stress and degree of ego strength.[4]

Dr. Bernard Rubin from the University of Chicago stated recently that, "the major mental illness rates are not comparable to violence rates and the distribution of major mental illness is not the same as the distribution of violence." Rubin concludes, "It is unlikely that dangerousness can be predicted in a person who has not acted in a dangerous or violent way. From a preventive point of view, it has been shown that gun control could reduce the number of fatalities resulting from acts of violence, but no body of knowledge about human behavior gives the information to make predictions about potential initial violence."[5]

The role of alcohol, drugs or other stimulants, or provocative social experiences cannot be discounted in the prediction of violent behavior. Aside from such organic or genetic influences as the XYY chromosome or temporal lobe epilepsy, which have been implicated in violent behavior, the newer syndrome entitled "episodic dyscontrol" is discussed by Dr. Barry Maletsky[6] who concludes that the twenty-two subjects he studied demonstrated,

> violent loss of this control upon minimal provocation, aurae and post-ictal states following such episodes, a history of alcoholism and increased aggression after alcohol, childhood history of hyperkinesis and truancy in a family background of alcoholism, sociopathy and violence in the males, and depression in the females. Such patients had frequently been in trouble with the law and were especially prone to use their automobiles aggressively. None of the twenty-two patients demonstrated obvious brain disease until adequately evaluated. Even after thorough examination (in most patients) brain abnormalities could not be absolutely documented in many patients. Nevertheless, the large majority responded to *Dilantin®*.

In another paper, Goldzband[7] defines dangerousness as, "the quality of an individual or a situation leading to the potential or actuation of harm to an individual, community or social order. It is inherent in this definition that dangerousness is not necessarily destructive (as destructive is commonly defined), although frequently seen as such by specific individuals or social orders threatened by such a quality."

Kozol, et al.[8] state clearly, "Dangerousness in criminal offenders can be reliably diagnosed and effectively treated with a recidivism rate of 6.1 percent." They define "dangerousness as a potential for inflicting serious bodily harm on another." They base their statements on a ten year study involving 592 male convicted offenders. They also conclude, "No tests or psychiatric examinations can dependably predict a probability of dangerous behavior in the absence of an actual history of a seriously violent assault on another person. The potential for dangerous behavior is relative and covers a wide spectrum, from the mildly dangerous to the extremely dangerous." They feel that the best treatment is psychiatric and discount the claims of others for the effectiveness of pharmacological or physiological treatment. They also found that their treatment methods were successful in modifying the dangerous potential of 94 percent of the patients. Finally they conclude, "It appears that dangerousness can be reliably diagnosed and effectively treated. It is clear that we must improve our diagnostic and therapeutic competence to ensure that fewer dangerous persons are let out and fewer nondangerous persons are kept in."

The adage, "violence breeds violence," is reflected by many violent individuals who have indicated that their fathers were brutal to them. Examples of beatings and merciless brutality to them as children are told often by prisoners. Excessive deprivation by parents occasionally leads to explosive violence in their children. In cases of parricide (killing of the parents by children) the parent who was killed repeatedly imposed violent, brutal conditions upon the child, who retaliated with explosive fury.[9]

One youngster from New Jersey who killed his father in a rage, described a life-long history of paternal abuse and cruelty, a history substantiated by his mother.

Many people who commit violent crimes have a history of emotional or physical trauma at an early age, e.g. an auto accident with resultant damage, or a long hospital stay with slow recovery, or other type of physical assault on the body that has been inadequately repressed. Often a history of a triad of firesetting, cruelty to animals, and enuresis is noted in the young child who later commits violent crimes. Can such behavior be prevented after we become aware of these syndromes? In essence, can we use preventive detention to "help" these youngsters?

In addition to emotional factors, organic conditions need to be explored. We have read about the XYY chromosome configuration in violent prisoners. It was seen in a significant number in those who had committed violent crimes, but is also seen in normals who do not commit violence and therefore cannot be a *sine qua non* to violent behavior. Hormonal and genetic changes may be significant factors. Mentally retarded individuals may commit crimes because they do not comprehend the communications of others.

We are in the process of evaluating a twenty-six-year-old man who periodically flies into a rage without apparent provocation. He has seriously harmed two policemen attempting to arrest him. He has had three abnormal EEG's. What is the relationship between his brain damage and his violent behavior? How significant are seizures in the perpetration of criminal and violent behavior? Psychomotor seizures; i.e. those in which the focus of the illness is in the temporal lobe, have been shown to be related to abrupt violent behavior.

The role of alcohol and drugs in lowering inhibition and creating confusion and clouding judgment needs to be mentioned as significant factors in the commission of crimes and the perpetration of violent behavior.

One of the most dangerous types of individuals is the paranoid schizophrenic who imagines or hallucinates, or has delusions that someone is after him. We need only look to early English legal history to the M'Naghten Case, where Daniel M'Naghten was suffering from the delusion that he was being persecuted by the Tories and felt he had to kill Sir Robert Peele, the prime minister of England, in 1843, in order to save himself. Or the Hadfield Case, in 1800, that Erskine defended so well, in which the defendant felt he had to kill in order to save mankind. These men are dangerous.

The law has maintained it is better for ten guilty men to go free in order to spare one innocent man from being incarcerated. In a contrary fashion we have over-included predictions of dangerousness so that one dangerous man will not go free; or it appears better to lock up ten who might be potentially violent than to let a dangerous man remain in the street to harm others. We must also consider the idea that many of these people who become criminals were also victims, victims earlier in life of tragedies that had befallen them. These tragedies may be parental rejection, serious emotional deprivation or physical injury. In an unpublished study by Dr. Joseph Peters at Philadelphia General Hospital, the victims of rape and sexual assault may reveal, on long-term follow-up, the effect of such sexual assault on the developing personality and future behavior of the victims.

Occasionally one may accurately predict the cause of violence in a youngster and be in a position to make specific recommendations to the parents for dealing with this aberrant behavior and curtail it.

> Several years ago the author saw a young divorced woman who revealed that her nine-year-old son was "burning up the hills of Santa Monica." In the course of the interview she was asked about sleeping arrangements and found that she shared her bed with her son. She was told to get her son his own bed in another room, and he would stop setting fires. On follow-up, after he had his own bed, he stopped lighting fires and became generally less anxious.

One other aspect of prediction that has emerged from experience is the notion that some people commit crimes in order to prevent themselves from becoming psychotic. The author has seen several young men who were aware that they were becoming mentally ill, and in an attempt to avoid the illness, acted out in criminal behavior. These men have admitted that they had chosen the legal means of obtaining help, rather than medical means because they were afraid of psychiatric treatment.[10]

Others have utilized criminal behavior as a means of masking mental illness and unless the illness is treated or controlled, the criminal behavior will continue. How convenient is the hippie subculture for the paranoid schizophrenic in which to lose himself. He can assume the guise of the hippie and maintain his bizarre ways, being seen only as different, rather than "crazy."

Many of these relationships may seem strange or contrived, and they certainly are not meant to be causal, one-to-one factors. By far the greater number of criminals are not seriously mentally ill; i.e. do not have a major mental illness, but may have characterological disorders, sociopathic tendencies or psychoneurotic traits. Only 25 percent of the inmates at Eastern State Penitentiary in Philadelphia, several years ago, were found to be suffering from major mental illness and psychosis, but were not sent to hospitals because they were not causing any trouble.

That many of our criminals are seriously mentally ill may be noted quite clearly in hospitals for the criminally insane that punctuate many of our states. These hospitals have recently come under notoriety following the *Baxstrom Decision*[11] releasing over nine hundred men. Psychiatrists have been instrumental in diagnosing people as seriously mentally ill and of criminal tendencies and recommend such hospitals as Matteawan State Hospital in New York, or Farview State Hospital in Pennsylvania. However, when we find upon release that these men are not dangerous or violent after several years at large, we begin to question our predictive abilities and our role in treating these men.

The youngsters who initially get into trouble with the law become arrested and labeled as criminally deviant, delinquent, unmanageable, incorrigible, etc. We know that many of these youngsters come from broken homes, fatherless homes, poor socioeconomic environments, have difficulty with truancy to avoid gang violence, and are immediately taken over by the authorities and labeled within the criminal subculture. Criminologists write about a subculture of violence where aggressive, violent behavior is encouraged by the group rather than discouraged as in middle class society. What we label criminal behavior may be necessary for survival in some subcultures.

Many people who emerge from the ghettos indicate that one has to live "by the law of the jungle" in order to survive. That usually means hustling, prostitution, drug peddling, all of which are crimes by our standards. In these people it is not difficult even for a nonpsychiatrist to predict criminal behavior. At the other extreme, we have the example of Charles Whitman, who told a psychiatrist that he felt like going up on the tower in Texas and killing a number of people. Many have criticized the psychiatrist for not reporting these fantasies or wishes that Whitman had prior to his eventual blood bath. Can the psychiatrist accurately predict when such a fantasy will be carried out? It is often very difficult to know when one is dealing with fantasy or "mere wishes" and whether these wishes will be acted upon in reality.

Furthermore, can a psychiatrist working in a prison help the parole board to know what men can safely be placed on parole without the extra risk of their committing further violent or nonviolent crimes? Or can a psychiatrist working in a hospital really know when a person has been "cured" or is well enough so that he can return to society without trying to take his own or someone else's life?

Two examples will illustrate the difficulties involved.

> The first case is a tragic one involving a malpractice suit in the midwest several years ago, where a young man was hospitalized because his wife was afraid that he was going to kill her. He never made any threats to the doctors in the hospital that he would do so, but his wife continued to fear for her life. The doctors treated this man in the hospital for several months until they felt he was ready to return to the community. When plans were made for his ultimate discharge on work release, so that he could live at the hospital and work at his old job, the communication of the fears of his wife to the employer was not made.
>
> The wife continued to protest, and the patient, instead of going to work, went immediately to his home and killed his wife.

Here is a glaring example in which the psychiatrists were fooled, were not able to predict that this man would go out and kill, and did not trust the pleadings of his desperate wife.

A second example of the type of predictions a psychiatrist must make in criminal situations emerges from a study that was conducted several years ago at the State Correctional Institution in Philadelphia.

> Several prisoners were selected by an experienced probation officer and divided into four different groups for the purpose of evaluating their state of dangerousness and prediction of future violent behavior. In the first group, a number of prisoners was selected who were deemed to be extremely dan-

gerous violent men by the warden. The second group was a number of inmates who were refused parole by the parole board because they were "not ready" for discharge; the third group was composed of those men who had been returned to prison because they had committed a violent violation of their parole, and the fourth group or "control group" were those men who had committed a technical or nonviolent violation of parole and returned to prison.

A thorough study of all groups indicated that most of the men emerged from fatherless or broken homes and had emotional or physical trauma in early childhood. The first group was composed primarily of the "con artists," the men who had caused trouble in prison, were not necessarily violent or dangerous men themselves, but were mostly psychopathic and would lead others to commit violence. The second group was considered extremely dangerous by the parole officer in his evaluation, though not necessarily so by the psychiatrist.

The third group was considered to be dangerous both by warden and parole officer because they had committed violent acts, and on the basis of their previous behavior were so labeled. The psychiatrist was not as concerned about the dangerousness in this group as was the warden and parole officer.

In the fourth group, both warden and parole officer felt the men were not necessarily violent but the psychiatrist, looking to ego strength and other psychodynamic factors found one or two whom he considered to be extremely dangerous men. Primarily, the prediction of future violent behavior or consideration of dangerousness was based upon the labeling and the selection of the men in the first place. Thus, there was a built-in bias to the study which indicated that the background and frames of reference of the evaluators contributed greatly to their prediction ability.

This study is presented as an example of the kinds of predictions that are made with reference to criminal behavior. It is wise that such predictions are not made by one man or one discipline, but by a number of men representing a variety of specialties. Each of the men would look for a different factor or different set of criteria in determining a man's readiness to take his place in society. If it were left up to the psychiatrist alone, he would make a number of errors because he would likely base his prediction primarily on what he is trained to observe, that is, internal psychodynamics rather than external behavior or circumstances, which are considered more important by sociologists, parole officers and correctional personnel. This study therefore demonstrates the differences that people use in predicting violence.

Some have said that the psychiatrist can more accurately predict future violent behavior if he has evidence that the individual already committed a crime or that he has been involved previously in violent behavior. A person who has committed violent acts previously may be more likely to do so again. The prediction becomes more accurate if this information is available to the psychiatrist. Some have insisted that the psychiatrist examine a person "cold" or "blindly," without the benefit of his past record.

However, the author utilizes all material available in making any kind of evaluation on a person involved in legal matters. A comprehensive evaluation from as many sources as possible is often helpful. These sources include relatives, spouse, people close at hand at the scene, any police reports and interviews with police officers who made up the reports. The psychiatrist who is asked to do this has become an investigator in the criminal-legal procedures and must utilize the predictive ability of other disciplines as well as his own. Fortunately, the disposition is determined by the judge and the psychiatrist merely gives an opinion and a recommendation. This recommendation cannot be based on traditional psychiatric methods alone. It must have included all available resources including criminological, sociological, statistical, psychological, medical and organic for the psychiatrist to pull together in his prediction.

Occasionally the psychiatrist does not have all this extra material at his disposal. He may be asked to examine and evaluate an individual who has committed a single crime and prepare a statement about the defendant's state of mind which led up to the crime, his subsequent response to the offense and a prediction within reasonable medical certainty whether such behavior would be likely to be repeated. This type of evaluation occurs most frequently in middle-class defendants who have committed a sexual offense, such as indecent exposure, indecent assault or sodomy; i.e. a homosexual act.

Often the history is that of a fairly compulsive, rigid individual who has not been able freely to express his sexual desires but who has maintained a facade of a "healthy life." Usually he is married, with a family, and occasionally is a professional person. Often he will deny that he was involved in the act for which he was accused, but later will admit with some degree of shame and remorse that he acted foolishly and impulsively.

In many of these cases the act of being caught, with its attendant stressful and anxiety-provoking experiences, is sufficient to prevent recurrence of the behavior. That is, the need to continue his good name in the community and his respect among his friends and relatives, with attendant feelings of guilt and shame, is sufficient to serve as a check against repeated impulsive behavior of that type.

Occasionally, however, we note a pattern of behavior which has proceeded undetected for several months or years. This usually involves the exhibitionist who has been "lucky" enough to get away with this behavior. Experiences he encounters when apprehended serve to keep him from recidivating temporarily, but when the pressure is eased there is great likelihood that he will repeat his pattern of behavior unless he receives appropriate psychotherapy.

One of the most difficult tasks of the forensic psychiatrist in this regard is to evaluate an ostensibly healthy individual who is accused of a homosexual act with a youngster. For example, the teacher who is accused of having homosexual experiences with one of his young adolescent pupils. The teacher denies this behavior and gives many good reasons why the youngster has cause to be angry with him and to bring such accusations against him. There is no confession; there is no indication on the part of the defendant that he has sexual problems which led up to the behavior in question. The psychiatrist is then asked to evaluate the defendant and tell the court that he is or is not likely to behave in such a manner and that he has or has not homosexual proclivities.

This is an extremely difficult task and often is beyond the scope of our expertise. Certainly we may evaluate a person and decide that he has sexual aberrations or deviations and psychological testing may be utilized to confirm or support our clinical impressions. However, to be able to state in the negative that after one or two visits, even with psychological testing, that the person has no tendency toward sexual aberration with the implication therefore that he could not have been involved in the act of which he is accused, borders on the speculative. It is wise to refrain from involving oneself in such communications.

The author offers the following experience.

A young, twenty-seven-year-old music teacher was accused by a fourteen-year-old male student of having indecent relations with him in the closet of the schoolroom on several occasions. The teacher denied his behavior and stated that the student was confused and angry, and wished to retaliate against the teacher for his not selecting him for one of the honors bestowed for that year. After several examinations of the defendant, who was a small, slight, rather effeminate looking individual, it was concluded that, despite his appearance, he did not seem to have homosexual propensities and was not likely to act out with a young male student. He denied his involvement and the author was asked to testify as an expert witness. Fortunately, the judge ruled that the testimony was not permissible in the case.

After the teacher was found guilty of his behavior, and given a probationary sentence, he admitted to his attorney that he had been involved and wished to set the record straight since the trial was over.

This is one area in which the psychiatrist may overstep his bounds as consultant and educator to the court and begin to assume the task left to the judge and/or jury. It is not the psychiatrist's function to determine whether a person did or did not commit an act (though the author has occasionally been asked this by a judge or a cross-examining attorney) but it is our role to clarify whenever we can, the mental state of an individual at a specific time within the criminal process.

Occasionally the psychiatrist is asked to examine an individual on a "one-shot" basis and prepare a report for forensic purposes. Sometimes this is possible and the situation is clear enough that such a report can be prepared, after an initial interview. However we have found that a series of interviews produces a much more valid and reliable result. In one study at Philadelphia General Hospital, we found that a series of group therapy sessions provides an even more reliable factor of prediction of future behavior than a single interview.[12]

What has been presented is a broad scope of the role of psychiatry in criminal procedures with reference to criminal psychodynamics, the ability of psychiatrists to predict in criminal matters dangerous or violent behavior. We do not have all the answers to the questions. What we need is to ask more questions, more sophisticated questions which will focus on more specific answers. We know generally where to look for what factors are involved, what syndromes, triads and symptoms are significant. Sometimes we can spot the symptoms in the youngster even before he becomes a criminal.

The question is, what do we do with this information once we have it? We need help from the law to be able to impose certain restrictions or effect treatment programs upon youngsters who demonstrate a need for help lest they become criminal or violent.

We need the kinds of institutions that can take care of people before they become trained criminals, and we also need institutions where we can rehabilitate our youngsters without making them "better" criminals. Many judges will put offenders on probation rather than into prison because they are afraid of what prison will do to these people, especially the youngsters, and trust the men on probation will be able to handle themselves fairly well, if given a chance. What they do not understand is that many probation officers are sorely overworked and cannot really control their probationers, nor are the necessary treatment resources available for adequate rehabilitation of probationers and parolees.

In summary, the psychiatrist is only one influence in the whole predictive mechanism of our legal correctional system. He offers the internal psychodynamic views to complement the behavioristic, statistical and phenomenological view of the correctional officer, probation officer and criminologist.

Predictions are often not accurate and refinements of techniques are sorely needed. Our youngsters in the precriminal population need guidance to keep them from criminal behavior. Those who have committed crimes are in need of effective rehabilitation to help keep them from becoming recidivists. This is truly a frontier area for law and psychiatry; it is vastly more important than any consideration of criminal insanity or competency to stand trial, both of which are essential in our criminal legal system.

Too much print and time has been spent on responsibility and competency, and precious little energy has been expended by lawyers and psychiatrists working together to help solve dispositional and prognostic predictive problems in the criminal law. Hopefully this imbalance will soon be corrected.

REFERENCES

1. Glueck, S., and Glueck, E.: *Unraveling Juvenile Delinquency.* Cambridge, Harvard U Pr, 1950.
2. Glueck, S., and Glueck, E.: *Predicting Delinquency and Crime.* Cambridge, Harvard U Pr, 1967.
3. Rappeport, J.: *The Clinical Evaluation of the Dangerousness of the Mentally Ill.* Springfield, Thomas, 1967.
4. Heller, M. S.: Dangerousness, diagnosis and disposition. Crime Commission of Philadelphia, Sentencing Institute, June, 1968.
5. Rubin, B.: Prediction of dangerousness in mentally ill criminals. *Arch Gen Psychiatry,* 27:397-407, Sept., 1972.
6. Maletsky, B.: The episodic dyscontrol syndrome. *Dis Nerv Syst,* March, 1973.
7. Goldzband, M.: On dangerousness. *Bull AAPL,* Dec., 1973.
8. Kozol, H., et al.: The diagnosis and treatment of dangerousness. *Crime and Delinquency,* October, 1972.
9. Sadoff, R. L.: Clinical aspects of parricide. *Psychiatr Q, 45:*65, 1971.
10. Sadoff, R. L.: Criminal behavior masking mental illness. *Corr Psychiat J Soc Ther,* 17:41, No. 2, 1971.
11. *Baxstrom v. Herold,* 383, US, 107, Feb., 1966.
12. Sadoff, R. L., Roether, H., and Peters, J. J.: Clinical measure of enforced group psychotherapy. *Am J Psychiatr, 128:*224, Aug., 1971.

Chapter 10

THE PSYCHIATRIST AND THE JUVENILE IN CRIMINAL PROCEEDINGS

IN MOST JURISDICTIONS the youthful offender is handled differently from the adult criminal. Every effort is made to keep the juvenile under the age of eighteen from obtaining a criminal record when he commits offenses. Most courts have a juvenile division in which special judges are assigned to handle the cases of juvenile delinquents, dependent or neglected children. A neglected child is one who is not properly cared for in his home and will need to be placed in an appropriate foster home or adoption institution. A dependent child is one who has not committed any offense but who becomes dependent upon the state by virtue of his inability to be cared for at home. Often he is also placed in an appropriate institution. The truant youngster or the runaway may be included in this category if no other offensive behavior is demonstrated.

Occasionally the juvenile will become involved in burglary, larceny, arson, malicious mischief, breaking and entering, assault and battery, incorrigibility, juvenile drinking or, increasingly more common, drug abuse. In all these instances the juvenile will be treated as a delinquent and not as a criminal. The rationale is that the state assumes the role of *parens patria* and the judge has a familial interest in the juvenile, not wishing to punish but to correct and rehabilitate.

The first juvenile court statute was enacted in Illinois in 1899, and subsequently every state has adopted one. The developers and authors of the statutes believed that society's role was not to determine whether a child was guilty or innocent, but as restated by the court to determine "what he is, how he has become what he is and what could best be done in his interest and in the interest of the state to save him from a downward career" (387,

U.S. 1, 15). The procedures for the treatment and rehabilitation were to be clinical rather than punitive.

Because the proceedings were not considered criminal, it was held that a juvenile was not entitled to bail, to indictment by a grand jury or to trial by jury. In adjudication, the child who was delinquent was not to have an effect of civil disability, or to be disqualified from civil service appointment.

These conditions in the juvenile courts were both substantive and operative until May 15, 1967, when the Supreme Court of the United States handed down the famed Gault Decision.[1] In essence that decision held that every constitutional protection afforded an adult, whether pretrial, at trial or post-trial, must be afforded the juvenile. Also, it stated that any treatment of the juvenile over and beyond the granting of these constitutional protections more favorable to him than corresponding treatment of adults will be favored. These constitutional protections included notice of the charges, right to be represented by counsel and constitutional privilege against self-incrimination.

The Gault Decision was based on the following set of circumstances.

On June 8, 1964, Gerald Gault, a fifteen-year-old boy, was arrested for making lewd or indecent remarks to a woman over the telephone. He was apprehended at 10:00 AM, while both his parents were at work. His parents were not advised of his arrest. Mrs. Gault learned later, through her own efforts, that Gerald was in the detention home and that the hearing would be held the following day in juvenile court. Mrs. Gault was present at the hearing but the lady who had received the obscene call was not present. No one was sworn nor was a transcript of the proceeding made. Gerald was questioned by the judge and there is conflict as to exactly what was said.

The hearing ended without a final decision but Gerald was detained until June 11 or 12. Four days later, further hearings were held with both Mr. and Mrs. Gault present. Again the complainant was not present and no record of the proceedings was made. At that time Gerald was under six months' probation for having been in the company of another boy who had stolen a wallet from a lady's purse.

When Gerald was arrested, another boy was in his presence, and Mrs. Gault wished the complainant to be present so it could be determined accurately which boy had made the obscene comments. Gerald would be committed to the state industrial school until age twenty-one, unless the institution discharged him sooner. In Arizona, under the Criminal Code, an adult with this offense would be subject to a fine of five dollars to fifty dollars, or imprisonment for not more than two months.

On appeal to the U.S. Supreme Court it was argued that Gerald Gault was taken from his parents without due process and that the following basic rights were denied.
1. notice of the charges
2. right to counsel
3. right to confrontation and cross-examination
4. privilege against self-incrimination
5. right to transcript of the proceedings
6. right to appellate review

The court agreed that the due process clause of the Fourteenth Amendment applied to minors and that Gerald indeed was denied his rights under the Constitution of the United States. The court reviewed the history of the theory of the juvenile court movement in which a child is made to feel that he is the object of the state's care and solicitude and not that he is under arrest or trial. However, the court noted the differential between theory and practice and said, "Unfortunately, loose procedures, high-handed methods and crowded court calendars, either singly or in combination, all too often have resulted in depriving some juveniles of fundamental rights that have resulted in a denial of due process."

The Gault Decision raised many questions from lawyers and courts as well as for juveniles. From a practical point of view it was impossible to overhaul the juvenile court system to meet the new requirements of this decision; for all practical purposes juvenile courts have not changed significantly because of this decision. However, if a juvenile demands a jury trial or if he demands a right to counsel, it is usually given him. Along with counsel, the juvenile also has a right to psychiatric examination and evaluation as does an adult under similar circumstances. One of the problems encountered is the proper disposition of the juvenile adjudged delinquent and in need of intensive care. There are very few adequate facilities to handle the emotionally disturbed juvenile delinquent. There are even fewer to handle the mentally retarded juvenile delinquent. State hospitals usually are not geared for such care and the juvenile is often sent to the "reform school," the county farm or the juvenile correctional institution.

The psychiatric role in criminal proceedings for juveniles is similar to the role the psychiatrist plays for adults, except that the insanity defense is rare and the bulk of psychiatric testimony is offered for dispositional recommendations.

The following case serves to illustrate the psychiatric and legal mechanisms involved in the adjudication of a juvenile accused of homicide.

> John is a twelve-year-old boy who was arrested for shooting his twenty-six-year-old brother with his mother's pistol during an argument at home. John had been reprimanded by his brother and his father on that day; during a physical altercation between John, his twelve-year-old boyfriend and John's brother, John went into his home, found the gun, loaded it, came out and threatened his brother. He said he only wanted to frighten him but his brother "Moved the wrong way" and was killed. John showed little remorse for what he had done, and tended to blame his brother's death on his brother's behavior. John assumed a vindictive, angry attitude toward everyone, especially his family. Following the shooting, he ran and hid for two days until he was later apprehended in the basement of his home.
>
> He was sent to the juvenile detention home where he was seen for psychiatric examination.
>
> John appeared to be an average size, blonde-haired lad who

seemed older than his stated age and presented his difficulties in a hostile, surly, challenging and vindictive manner. During the course of the examination he became docile, cooperative and friendly. However, when discussing his family and especially his mother, father and brother, his defensiveness rose to the surface.

During one visit, when he was interviewed with his mother, he became extremely hostile and aggressive toward her, with irrational thought processes. He later calmed down and apologized for his erratic and irrational behavior. He was seen to be an escape risk and the custodians at the detention center were advised of this opinion. John did escape from the detention home on at least one occasion before his hearing.

Psychological testing revealed that John was suffering from an ego defect, was basically schizoid, with predisposition for schizophrenic decompensation under appropriate stress. An insanity defense was not offered, nor would it have been helpful in this case. Primarily in adult cases, the insanity defense is offered to keep the defendant from being executed in capital offenses. There is no capital punishment for juveniles in Pennsylvania.

John could be incarcerated only until he was twenty-one, unless reevaluation at the age of twenty-one revealed that he required further hospital care and would be civilly committed by the court.

In juvenile cases the probation officer is an important advisor to the court, and in this situation the juvenile's attorney, his probation officer, the examining psychiatrist and the judge all worked together to effect an optimal disposition for John. All recognized that he was seriously emotionally disturbed and most likely had been mentally ill at the time of the shooting, and that he continued to be potentially dangerous under appropriate stressful conditions.

The recommendation was for inpatient treatment in a state hospital setting, with gradual release to the community when he was no longer considered dangerous. Preliminary exploration of the state hospitals revealed that none in the vicinity had facilities to handle John's problems. It was felt that a minimum security correctional institution such as a boy's farm or a forestry camp would not be suitable for him. It was finally decided that a special school for boys with emotional problems and acting out behavior was available and would be able to accept John as a resident.

From a legal point of view, a *prima facie* case had to be made out for homicide in the court record. After the *prima facie* case was made, petition for transfer of the case to juvenile court was made to try the youngster as a juvenile rather than as an adult. Once in juvenile court and examination and evaluation of the facts of the case was conducted in order to determine the guilt or innocence of the defendant and degree of homicide. Later a hearing to determine disposition was conducted. From a practical point of view, these procedures occurred consecutively on the same day, with the psychiatrist testifying at all three in one sitting. First, the psychiatrist testified that the juvenile was immature and emotionally ill and should not be tried as an adult because of his youth and his inexperience. Next, when the case was remanded to the juvenile court, the psychiatrist continued his testimony regarding the state of mind of the youngster at the time of the shooting, indicating that he was seriously emotionally disturbed and mentally ill. He then testified to disposition, recommending hospitalization for a long period of time for intensive treatment with medication.

At a subsequent hearing, following the exploration of facilities available, the psychiatrist returned to testify about the optimal institution for this youngster. At the hearing, respresentatives of each of the institutions to which the youngster could be referred were present to discuss with the judge facilities available for comprehensive treatment and rehabilitation. When the institution of choice was decided upon, the judge made a personal trip to the home before sending the boy there.

This is an unusual case which is presented to highlight many of the areas in juvenile criminal proceedings which do not occur in the adult courts. Homicide by a twelve-year-old is rare. Usually when a juvenile of fifteen or sixteen commits a homicide he is tried as an adult and is punished as one, rather than given the benefits of the juvenile court proceedings. In this instance, however, the immaturity and youthfulness of the defendant warranted against an adult proceeding. It should be noted that he was represented by counsel, and the district attorney was able to cross-examine all witnesses. The judge had taken a special interest in the case and worked cooperatively with the district attorney, the probation officer, the defense counsel and the psychiatrist, first in making a determination of the commission of the crime, secondly the guilt or innocence of the defendant and, most importantly, the final disposition. This case is unique also in that it consumed many hours of professional time and was not handled "routinely" or with dispatch. All legal safeguards and constitutional rights of the defendant were upheld while he was given the best opportunity available for future recovery.

It should be noted on follow-up that while John was being detained pending the judge's return from visiting the institution to which he was to be committed, he escaped from the juvenile home. He was a fugitive for two years in the area. Typically, upon apprehension the judge would have sentenced the youngster to a maximum security institution for juveniles because of his escape and his potential dangerousness. However, the judge found that during the two years that John was away no violence occurred and there was found, at subsequent psychiatric examination, to be potential for growth, maturation and acceptance of social norms. The judge placed the boy in a suitable foster home and follow-up evaluation shows no further episodes of violence.

Discussion of this case and management in juvenile court leads to a subtopic of juvenile crime which is of some significance. This is the crime of parricide—the killing of one's parents. The following chapter is a republication of a previous article that appeared in the *Psychiatric Quarterly*, in 1971. It is presented to provide the reader with clinical evidence for psychodynamic factors in the killing of one's parents by juveniles.

REFERENCES

1. *Gault v. Ariz.* 387, U.S. 1, May, 1967.

Chapter 11

CLINICAL OBSERVATIONS ON PARRICIDE

FREUD PRESENTED the original psychodynamic considerations on parricide and noted that three of the masterpieces of literature of all time, *Oedipus Rex*, of Sophocles, Shakespeare's *Hamlet*, and Dostoevsky's *The Brothers Karamazov*, all deal with this subject.[1] Wertham coined the term "Orestes Complex" based on the Greek play in which Orestes returns to kill his mother to avenge his father's murder.[2] In all cases, the subject is depicted as mad or mentally ill and in Freud's references, sexual rivalry for a woman appears to be the principal motivating factor. Wertham describes a clinical entity he calls "catathymic crisis": the killing is a result of the building up of unconscious tension due to external situational pressures, for which there appears no other alternative but violence. Provocation, if present at all, is usually insignificant. The killer usually blames the external situation for his internal tension and holds the victim responsible for his act.

Vereecken credits Asselin for the following observation made in 1901. "There is no question of malice aforethought, parricide is committed in a sudden fit of rage, there is no choice of weapon." In his review of the literature, Vereecken found, "the diversity of characteristics of a mental disorder is great in the literature in cases of parricide."[3]

Mecir presents a series of child murderers including six involving parents, and notes, "Murder was perpetrated in a state of severely altered mental condition where the criminal has completely lost control over his actions and is incapable of realizing there is social danger."[4] Stutte, in studying an attempted parricide by a sixteen-year-old girl, found that the,

---

Originally published in modified form in *Psychiatric Quarterly*, 45:65-69, No. 1, 1971.

... dispositional, constellational and situational components of the act are devoid of extraordinary dramatic or conflictual crises. Also, with full knowledge of the girl's personality structure, family situation and actual state before the act, an expert could hardly have predicted such a vehement and dangerous outburst of emotion. Such potential reactions are, as this case shows, continually present in normal adolescents in conflict situations typical for the developmental stage.[5]

In a thirty year study of 122 homicide cases admitted to the Ontario hospital, twelve were cases of matricide. The authors found that both matricide and patricide are rare occurrences and they are virtually always carried out by the sons. Matricide was found to be more frequent than patricide.[6] Morris found twenty matricides in a study of 245 family murders; of these, nineteen mothers were killed by their sons and one by a daughter. In the same group there were ten patricides; of these, nine fathers were killed by sons and one by a daughter.[7]

In a rather comprehensive article, O'Connell reviewed thirteen cases of matricide in a five year period, in Great Britain. The following characteristics were found to be significant. All of the killers were unmarried (one had had an unsatisfactory marriage), none had mature sexual feelings and the majority had overt homosexual contacts. Most had shown a close and excessive interest in their mother's sexual behavior. On the whole, they were characterized as passive-dependent, unambitious, hypochondriacal with strong feelings of sexual and social inferiority.

The precipitating cause was trivial or absent, but in five it involved separation from the mother. Eleven were diagnosed as schizophrenic and two as depressive. After the crime, most showed relief rather than distress or remorse; eleven later came to express regret and yearning.[8]

Raizen presents a case of matricide in which the killer is found to have a long-standing emotional disorder, overt homosexuality, gross attempts at sexual seduction on the part of the mother and a diagnosis of paranoid schizophrenia.[9] MacDonald reports in detail a case of a married male with hostile dependency toward his mother from whom separation caused him to kill her.[10]

CASE PRESENTATIONS

Two cases of parricide (one matricide, one patricide) occurred within the same county within the same year, having similar psychodynamics. Both killers were examined initially on the same day and revealed striking similarities in their psychodynamic difficulties.

Case Number One

John is a seventeen-year-old boy who was raised in a rural county and attended school in a small nearby town. He had had a great deal of difficulty in school and had been suspended on two or three occasions for stealing and lying. Each time he was suspended he was restricted to his room. The restrictions created further rebellious behavior, which resulted in further restrictions. John had been restricted almost consistently to his room for three to four years prior to his shooting his mother.

On the day of the killing he returned home early, on suspension from school for driving a friend's car in the school parking lot without permission. His mother scolded him, threatened him and said she would not care if his father killed him when he came home. She told him to stay where she could keep an eye on him and not to wander off. He had chores to do, one of which entailed going some distance from the house into the fields. He returned to the house to tell his mother that he needed to leave the immediate vicinity of the house and wished her to know. When he entered the house he saw his father's gun on the gun shelf, with shells nearby. Without saying anything, he picked up the gun, loaded it and began to fire at his mother, who was standing at the top of the stairs, holding one of the foster children who lived in their home. He ran up the stairs, continued to fire, having no later recall for his behavior.

He next recalled finding himself outside with the gun in his hand and hearing his mother screaming. He hurried up the stairs to see her lying in a pool of her own blood, and the three-year-old foster child was wounded. He immediately dialed the operator for the police and waited outside for the other foster children to return home for lunch, which he was planning to prepare for them. He was not aware that his mother was dead, but had some awareness that he must have shot her because the gun was in his hand.

His immediate reaction was one of relief, with no guilt or remorse. Following his relief, he felt depression at his behavior, especially because his father became mentally ill, had to be hospitalized and would have nothing to do with him. After six months in prison, awaiting trial, his depression was relieved.

Past History indicates that John was the older of two children, having a younger sister who was always favored by their mother, according to John and others. He described his having to work all day for little money, which he had to give to his mother for safekeeping. When he wanted the money to spend, his mother told him it was gone. However, his sister, who did not work, would always have money available to her when she wished. He grew up feeling that his mother was unfair to him.

His further frustrations were compounded by his mother taking in as many as twelve to fifteen foster children at a time, having four or five young boys under the age of five to share John's bedroom. It was his duty in the mornings to change the boys' diapers and give them breakfast before he went to school. He had no privacy in his home; he was restricted at home and not allowed to have treats at school. He began to steal and to save money that he had earned to put it in his locker in school.

John indicated that he got along fairly well with his father, whom he felt was trying to be fair to him, but who was dominated by his mother. He had tried to run away from home on several occasions but was unsuccessful, once because he became ill, and another time because of a heavy snowfall.

Following his incarceration, John had difficulty sleeping and had fantasies that his mother had not died. He had the impression that she was alive and he would go into the street and find her. He had dreams of going home and having his father trying to shoot him. He would visualize in his dream his father standing over him with a gun and pulling the trigger, only to find that it did not fire. His mother then would come out and laugh, saying it was only a joke and "it didn't work." He also had hypnagogic experiences in which he heard his mother calling his name for several days following the shooting. Later, after reconstituting in the prison, John said that he regrets in a way that his newfound relief and freedom had to come at the expense of his mother's life. He said he felt more like other children now that she was gone, whereas previously he felt different and not a part of his own society.

John indicated that two months prior to the shooting he felt that his thoughts were becoming confused and he requested from his mother to see a doctor about his problems. She refused him and his confusion increased.

Following further examination of John's mental state, including comprehensive psychological testing, it was determined that he was suffering from a serious depressive reaction which culminated in an acute psychotic episode at the time of the shooting. Since he showed no evidence for hallucinations or psychotic thought process at the time of the examination, six months after the shooting, it is difficult to establish a diagnosis of schiophrenic reaction for the period of his acute psychotic episode. However, psychological testing revealed that he had an underlying ego deficiency with schizoid adjustment. The psychiatric testimony was fairly consistent at time of trial regarding his psychodynamics and diagnosis. Differences occurred in applying the psychiatric findings to the test of insanity (McNaghten Rule). Despite conflicting testimony, John was acquitted on the basis of temporary insanity.

Case Number Two

Frank is a twenty-two-year-old single, concert pianist who shot and killed his father following an argument at a department store in a large suburban shopping center. The family had been on vacation and Frank had been frightened of his father and the guns that his father kept at home. He had tried unsuccessfully to get rid of his father's guns in the past and had taken one to the lake to throw it away. However, he was afraid that his father would become enraged when he returned home to find his gun missing. Hence, Frank attempted to bring the gun back secretly and replace it without his father's awareness. On the last leg of their return home, Frank had taken the gun from under the car seat and placed it in his pocket.

While in the store, Frank's father had berated him for being "no good as a worker, worthless and not entitled to a record" (that Frank wished to purchase). His father began choking Frank, saying he was going to kill him.

Frank broke loose and shot his father several times. According to witnesses, Frank shouted at his father as he shot him, "You won't hurt my mother any more." He was not aware of the shooting or his statement, did not hear the gun shots and awoke to find himself outside with no gun in his hands. Because he remembered last being in the store, with his parents, he returned to find people crouching behind counters and lying flat on the floor. He saw his father lying on the floor and attempted to go to him and kiss him but was restrained by his mother.

He was not aware that he had killed his father, and had hoped that his father would not die. After he was told that his father had died, Frank stated he felt relief and said, "I'm not afraid any more."

Past History reveals that Frank was born with a twin who was mentally retarded and required institutional care. At age four, Frank was sent to live in a foster home because his mother was needed to work when his father became mentally ill. At age eleven or twelve he returned to live with his parents because his father said, "He's now old enough to take care of himself." Frank's father had a serious problem with his temper and the family was afraid of him. Frank's mother did not leave her husband because she was afraid he would kill her if she did. Frank recalls his interest in playing the piano dating back to a very early age and his father's encouragement. Frank would be able to make enough money to support the family when his father was too old to work. Frank says he was always afraid of his father and could not understand why his father mistreated him for, he would do anything for his father.

His father would not forgive errors and would not apologize for his own. Frank said, "He would slap me, beat me, holler at me, tell me I'm not good for anything." Frank would then need to prove to his father that he was good at something. He recalls once when he was unable to play the piano because he had injured his finger, his father yelled at him and Frank ran from the house. He said he could not leave his father because his father needed him to help with his business. When he finally returned, his father made him get down on his knees, yelled at him, called him stupid, dragged him across the floor by his hair and said, "Stay down there like an animal." Frank recalls that his father was frequently beating his mother and when he tried to intervene, he also was beaten by his father.

Frank's mother related that her husband made Frank load one of the guns and then took it with his handkerchief so that Frank's fingerprints would be on the gun. If anything happened with that gun, i.e. if Frank and his mother were killed, the police would think Frank killed his mother and then himself. That was the gun that Frank used on his father. Frank's father also made him give up a girl friend that he liked very much because she would keep him from his career and deprive the family of Frank's income. Frank said later, "I could not let anything interfere with making my father happy."

On initial examination Frank revealed evidence of anxiety depression and active hallucinations with obsessive fears. His fingers would constantly move on any flat surface while he was talking and he indicated that he was practicing his musical scales. While describing the shooting, Frank recreated the scene in a most bizarre, trance-like manner, stating, "I'll make it up to you Papa, I'll be a success for you, Papa, why did you have to threaten me, Papa." When talking about his desire to kiss his father after the shooting, he said, "I never kissed my father."

Comprehensive psychological testing revealed that Frank had various underlying turbulence and turmoil, as reflected in the Rorschach Test. He was given a diagnosis by testing of schizophrenic reaction, paranoid type. His responses were bizarre and unusual, reflecting a psychotic condition. Subsequent clinical evaluation revealed that Frank had reintegrated and his bizarre behavior had abated.

Frank was released on bail and was seen as an outpatient. He began to work effectively and lived by himself, making new friends. He was seen to have a borderline psychotic state. It was also felt that at the time of the shooting he had experienced an acute psychotic deterioration, paranoid schizophrenic type, with "homosexual panic." Following the shooting, he felt relief, little remorse and a sense of freedom for the first time in his life. He regretted that his freedom had come at the price of his father's death, but he was pleased that he had his liberation.

He was seen by psychiatrists for the state, who had a similar evaluation of his mental status and also indicated that he had an altered state of consciousness at the time of the shooting. A pretrial agreement allowed Frank to plead guilty to voluntary manslaughter for which he would be sent for treatment for an indeterminate period of time.

Discussion

Both cases reveal many similar psychodynamics and family dynamics. Most striking is the cruel and unusual relationship between victim and assassin. Also, the bond that existed between child and parent was a dramatically ambivalent one of fear and hatred, on the one hand, and an inexplicable loyalty and yearning on the other. Neither child could leave the family, neither could free himself of the bond voluntarily and without explosive violence. Evidence of latent homosexuality was not as obvious in John as it was in Frank. In both cases the predictability of such violence was high, and relatives and friends, aware of the charged atmosphere, had warned the families of impending explosion if the relationships did not change.

On the basis of these two cases, coupled with a review of the literature on parricide, it may be concluded that a bizarre neurotic relationship exists between the victim and his assassin, in which the parent-victim mistreats the child excessively and pushes him to the point of explosive violence. The child is unable to leave voluntarily without such explosion due to a strong attachment to the opposite parent. A sense of relief rather than remorse or guilt is felt following the parricide, leading to a feeling of freedom from the abnormal relationship. As in other reported cases, the provocation may have been insignificant or similar to previous encounters that did not lead to such violence.

In the two cases reported a borderline or schizoid personality preexisted the acute psychotic deterioration at time of the shooting and the psychosis cleared following the act. In both instances the psychotic illness was most likely acute paranoid schizophrenic reaction which remitted spontaneously without medication. Also, in both cases as in previously reported cases, an altered state of consciousness existed at the time of the killing, with resultant later amnesia for the episode.

In these cases the availability of the guns played a most significant role as the weapon chosen for such explosive violence. It is unlikely in either case that an alternative weapon would have been as effective even if available. In one case the parent provided the weapon of his own destruction.[11, 12]

From a forensic psychiatric standpoint, both killers were given intensive psychiatric examinations by prosecution and defense. Juries and judges were found to be lenient and made every effort to understand the killing as resulting from serious intra-familial and intra-psychic conflicts. Accordingly, Vereecken summarizes the psychodynamics in his case of parricide as follows. "There is often a question of a dependent relationship toward a hatred authoritarian father, accompanied by an incestuous fixation upon the mother."[3]

In attempting to understand the psychodynamics of parricide, Freud initially discusses the Oedipal conflict within the boy in relation to his father.

> In addition to the hate which seeks to get rid of the father as a rival, a measure of tenderness for him is also habitually present. The two attitudes of mind combine to produce identification with the father; The boy wants to be in his father's place because he admires him and wants to be like him, and also because he wants to put him out of the way. This whole development comes up against a powerful obstacle. . . . The boy understands that he must also submit to castration if he wants to be loved by his father as a woman. Thus both impulses, hatred of the father, and being in love with the father, undergo repression. There is a certain psychological distinction in the fact that the hatred of the father is given up on account of fear of an external danger (castration), while the being in love with the father is treated as an internal instinctual danger, though fundamentally it goes back to the same external danger.[1]

The acting out of deep-rooted forbidden fantasies often leads to feelings of guilt and remorse. However, in the case of parricide, it appears that such explosive impulsive behavior leads more to feelings of relief from the bond that entrapped its victim. One reason put forth for this relief and lack of remorse is that the killer often blames the victim for setting up the circumstances of his own demise. Many have said, as in the case of the two patients reported here, that the parents killed themselves, using their sons as the weapon. It is this firm conviction on the part of the patient, or killer, supported by family members and others who were witness to the cruelty perpetrated by the victim upon the killer, that serves to release the guilt and allow the feeling of freedom and relief. Although this is a subjective feeling of the child who kills his parent, it would be teleological reasoning to insist that the parent actually committed suicide in this bizarre manner.

Summary

Two cases of parricide, one matricide, one patricide, are presented to illustrate the psychodynamic and forensic implications involved. A review of the literature supports the findings in these cases and reveals the explosive, often psychotic, reaction involved, with resultant feeling of relief and freedom following an initial depressive reaction.

REFERENCES

1. Freud, S.: Dostoevsky and parricide. *Collected Papers,* New York, Basic, 1959, vol. 5, p. 222.
2. Wertham, F.: *Dark Legend.* New York, Duell, 1941.
3. Vereecken, J. L.: A case of parricide. *Psychother Psychosom, 13:*364-79, 1965.
4. Mecir, J.: Homicidal behavior of minors directed against their parents. *Cesk Psychiatr, 64:*5, 1968.
5. Stutte, H.: Attempted parricide by a sixteen year old girl. *Acta Paedopsychiatr* (Basel), *31:*95-9, March, 1964.
6. McKnight, C. K., Mohr, J. W., Quinsey, R. E., and Erochko, J.: Matricide and mental illness. *Can Psychiatr Assoc J, 11:*99-106, 1966.
7. Morris, T., and Bloom-Coper, L. J.: Murder in microcosm. *The Observer,* 1961.

8. O'Connell, B. A.: Matricide. *Lancet,* 7290, May, 1963.
9. Raizen, K. H.: A case of matricide-patricide. *Br J Delinquency, 10:*4, 1960.
10. Macdonald, J. M.: *The Murderer and His Victim.* Springfield, Thomas, 1961.
11. Rotenberg, L. A., and Sadoff, R. L.: Who should have a gun? Some preliminary psychiatric thoughts. *Am J Psychiat, 125:*841, Dec., 1968.
12. Rotenberg, L. A., and Sadoff, R. L.: On guns: History, dynamics and control. *Corr Psychiat and J of Soc Therapy,* Winter, 1970.

Chapter 12

SEXUALLY DEVIATED OFFENDERS

EXAMINATION AND COMPARISON of the "sexual deviate" and the "sexual offender" as defined respectively by psychiatry and the law indicate vast differences in concepts and methods of application. Psychiatry "designates as sexual deviations or perversions, any patterns of sexual behavior which differ from normal coitus and serve as major sources of sexual gratification rather than as foreplay to coital activity."[1] Karpman refers to the sexually deviated individual as a paraphiliac and sees in him "profound disturbances in the sex life . . . and patterns of sexual behavior not directed ultimately toward procreation, the goal of all normal sex life."[2] Among the major sexual perversions or deviations listed in the *American Handbook of Psychiatry* are included overt homosexuality, pedophilia, fetishism, transvestitism, exhibitionism, voyeurism, sadomasochism, lust-murder, zoophilia, coprophilia and necrophilia.[1]

Differences in terminology and classification between sexual "deviates" and "offenders" are well illustrated by comparing the above list of sexual deviations with the list of offenses Pennsylvania considers to be sexual offenses: indecent assault, incest, assault with intent to commit sodomy, sodomy, assault with intent to ravish or rape, threat of bodily harm and mental harm.*

This chapter is reprinted with permission from the *Temple Law Q.*, Phila., Pa., USA, Vol. 40, Nos. 3-4, pp. 305-315, Spring-Summer, 1971.

* Barr-Walker Act, *Pa. Stat. Ann.* tit. 19, §1166 (1964). For the better administration of justice and the more efficient punishment, treatment and rehabilitation of persons convicted of the crime of indecent assault, incest, assault with intent to commit sodomy, sodomy, assault with intent to ravish or rape, if the court is of the opinion that any such person, if at large, constitutes a threat of bodily harm to members of the public, or is an habitual offender and mentally

(Continued on page 128)

Both lists refer to abnormal behavior of a sexual nature. Under the general offenses of indecent assault and sodomy may fall all sexual deviations involving another person. "Private" deviations such as transvestitism, fetishism and coprophilia are not covered by law unless larceny, burglary or other crime is committed in order to engage in the perversion. For example, a man may need to steal women's garments in order to dress up as a female and usually has a need to steal the object of his fetish, most commonly a piece of women's wearing apparel.

The law has tended to lump all individuals committing crimes involving sex into one group of criminals called sex offenders, or more recently, sexual psychopaths. Since 1938 more than half the states and the District of Columbia have passed so-called "sexual psychopath statutes," aimed at the protection of society and the rehabilitation of the offender. These laws have placed all sexual offenders into the class "sexual psychopath," in that they have imposed indeterminate sentences on the individual at the same time providing for treatment and rehabilitation within a prison or hospital facility.*

The major difficulty with these laws is that they have put a variety of types of individuals into a single classification with the intention of providing uniform or standard treatment for all. In many cases group psychotherapy, individual psychotherapy or counseling is recommended without the benefit of preliminary psychiatric evaluation. Such recommendation is based primarily on the commission of the abnormal sexual act constituting the sexual offense.

The American Bar Foundation, in its comprehensive study of 1961, attacks these sexual psychopath statutes for their improper classification.

---

ill, the court, in lieu of the sentence now provided by law, for each crime, may sentence such person to a State institution for an indeterminate term having a minimum of one day and a maximum of his natural life. On June 17, 1967 the sentencing aspect of this Act was held unconstitutional by the Pennsylvania Superior Court in *Commonwealth v. Dooley*—Pa. Super.—232 A. 2d 45 (1967). Revisions are currently under consideration. See *Philadelphia Evening Bulletin*, July 10, 1967, p. 9, col. 1.

* See e.g. *Pa. Stat. Ann.* tit. 19, §§1166-73 (Supp. 1966).

A major function of any law is to define clearly that class of persons to which the law applies. In this respect the sex deviate laws have failed. Although in some twenty-seven jurisdictions purport to deal with the same personality in their sex deviate laws, there are twenty-eight different definitions or descriptions of that personality.† From the psychiatric point of view, this is an extremely important criticism, as the term "psychopath" is too vague and general to be meaningful or useful. "The expression 'psychopath' is not a proper, adequately descriptive, or sufficiently explanatory medical term, nor is it diagnostically or dynamically acceptable. Its use as a legal definition, under the guise of a medical diagnosis, is particularly unfeasible."[3]

In 1950 the Group for the Advancement of Psychiatry cautioned "against the use of this appellation 'psychopath' in the law on several grounds. There is still little agreement on the part of psychiatrists as to the precise meaning of the term. Furthermore, the term has no dynamic significance."* In its revision of the psychiatric nomenclature, the American Psychiatric Association discarded the term "psychopathic personality" in favor of "personality disorder," which includes, among other categories, the "sociopathic personality disturbances."[4] The "sexual deviations" fall into this category as do the "antisocial reactions."

Following examination of three hundred sexual offenders, Ellis and Brancale concluded that ". . . legal designations and classifications of sex offenders were found to be quite confused, illogical, and overlapping, and to have little relationship to scientific classifications of these offenders."‡ They have suggested the following classification, now being utilized in the New Jersey Diagnostic Center.

A. Normal sex offenders, who are not sexual deviates but who commit illegal sex acts.
B. Sex deviates who commit illegal sex acts but who are sufficiently stable and well integrated to maintain their devia-

---

† *The Mentally Disabled and the Law* 305 (Lindman & McIntyre eds. 1961).
* Group for the Advancement of Psychiatry, Psychiatrically Deviated Sex Offenders (Report No. 19. 1950).
‡ Ellis and Brancale, *The Psychology of Sex Offenders* 93 (1956).

tional patterns without usually getting into official difficulties.

C. Sexually and psychiatrically deviated offenders who commit illegal sex acts and who are so emotionally disturbed or mentally impaired that they frequently come to official attention.

D. Psychiatrically but sexually nondeviated offenders, who commit illicit sex acts because of their general rather than their sexual disturbances, and who are often officially apprehended.‡

This four-part classification of sex offenders is significant in its recognition of the various types of individuals who may commit sex offenses and come to official attention. Many sex offenders may not be sexual deviates. They may be treatable deviates or sexual deviates whose behavior is difficult to control and who are therefore in need of institutionalization. Or they may be nonsexually deviated but emotionally disturbed and in need of treatment and/or institutionalization. This type of classification is geared toward prognosis, treatment and management of sex offenders and is not content with mere labeling and incarcerating as are many of the sexual psychopath statutes.

It is well recognized that the enactment of the sexual psychopath laws in many instances has been a hurried response to a public demand to "do something" about the "sex fiends" that are roaming the country. The laws provide for commitment but often do not specify where the commitment is to take place. Treatment has been provided for in the law but not in the community.

Much of the difficulty behind the errors in the handling of the sex offender may be traced to society's attitudes about sex and sexual misbehavior. Tappan lists eleven popular myths concerning sex offenders, including the notions that sex offenders are usually recidivists; that the minor sex offender, if unchecked, progresses to more serious types of crime; that it is possible to predict the danger of serious crimes by sexual deviates; that "sex psychopathy" or sex deviation is a clinical entity; that rea-

---

‡ *Ibid.*, pp. 93-94.

sonably effective treatment methods to cure deviant sex offenders are known and employed; and that the sex problem can be solved merely by passing a new law.*

Guttmacher and Wiehofen propose that four widely held misconceptions have been responsible for most of the defects in the laws passed to handle sex offenders.

a. Sex offenders are unique from other offenders.
b. Minor sex offenders later become major sex offenders.
c. Sex offenses are increasing in frequency.
d. All sex offenders are recidivists.†

The most important misconception seems to be the one that regards all sex offenders as belonging to the same group or classification. It is fallacious to group biological disorders together simply because they show one symptom. It is an error from the

---

* Tappan, "Some Myths About the Sex Offender," *Fed Prob* 19:7-12 (1955). See also the following comment from Mohr, Turner and Jerry, *Pedophilia and Exhibitionism* 85 (1964). The data point out that recidivism in sexual offenses is low in general. Exhibitionism has consistently the highest recidivism rate, followed by homosexual pedophilia with a recidivism rate from 13 percent to 28 percent. Heterosexual offenses against children show about half this recidivism rate, varying from 7 percent to 13 percent.

The chances of repeating the offense increase drastically with the number of convictions. In all sexual offenses, the chances of repeating the offense increase from about 10 percent for first offenders, to one out of three cases of previous sexual convictions and one out of two in cases of previous sexual and nonsexual convictions.

† Guttmacher and Weihofen, *Psychiatry and the Law* 111-12 (1952). In the first place, sex offenders are treated as if they comprise a separate and homogeneous group of criminals. The reverse is true. There is as much difference between the average exhibitionist and the average rapist as there is between the shoplifter and the safe-cracker. Secondly, it is believed that sex offenders regularly progress from minor offense such as exhibitionism to major offenses like forced rape. Such a graduation is almost unknown. The exhibitionist is acting out in an intrapsychic conflict. He has adopted this method of relieving an intolerable state of anxiety and tension. Paradoxically this has worked satisfactorily for him and he could not be induced to try a substitute. Then there is a widespread belief that sex offenses are rampant today, there has been a sudden alarming increase in their incidence. All of the careful investigations made recently have failed to demonstrate any persistent trend in that direction. A fourth major source of error is the belief that all sex offenders tend to be recidivists. In the last of the "Uniform Crime Reports" available, rape was twenty-third and "other sex offense" twenty-sixth in order of recidivism among the twenty-seven offenses listed.

medical viewpoint to group sex offenders under one diagnostic category although it may be feasible from a legal standpoint. Sex offenders are found among many diagnostic categories, some of which are the following: schizophrenia, schizoid personality disorder, psychoneurosis, psychopathic personality disorder, alcoholism, chronic brain syndrome, and mental defective.‡

Gray and Mohr summarize the difficulties in the classification of sex offenders by pointing out the inconsistencies involved in legal and medical labels for individuals who commit various offenses.§ Guttmacher and Weihofen describe as a general offender the emotionally disturbed individual whose difficulties may manifest themselves in isolated sexual offenses. They state that this individual should not be classified as a sexual offender.*

---

‡ Of the first three hundred convicted sex offenses seen at the New Jersey Diagnostic Center, the following frequency distribution of the diagnostic categories was found: Normal 14 percent; Mildly Neurotic, 29 percent; Severely Neurotic, 35 percent; Borderline Psychotic, 8 percent; Psychotic, 2 percent; Organic Brain Impairment, 5 percent; Psychopathic, 3 percent; Mentally Deficient, 4 percent. Ellis and Brancale, *The Psychology of Sex Offenders* 93 (1953), table 7, at 46.

§ Gray and Mohr, *in Sexual Behavior and the Law*, Slovenko, ed. (Springfield, Thomas, 1965). The task of identifying nosological groups which account for legal as well as clinical exigencies is complicated by the divergence of legal charges and clinical symptoms. Sexual deviations such as some forms of transvestism and fetishism may not constitute criminal offenses and a sexual offense, such as rape, especially statutory rape, may not denote a sexual deviation. A charge such as indecent assault may comprise sexually deviant acts arising from pedophilic impulses as well as sexual non-deviant acts such as accosting a woman in a park with "normal" sexual aims. Nonsexual offenses such as arson, theft and trespassing may arise out of deviant sexual impulses. Also, various acts representing one sexual deviation may be prosected under a variety of criminal charges. A pedophile, for instance, may be charged with indecent exposure, indecent act, indecent assault, lewd behavior with a minor, contribution to juvenile delinquency, attempted carnal knowledge or statutory rape and gross indecency.

* Guttmacher and Weihofen, *Psychiatry and the Law* 112-13 (1952). It is important to realize that some individuals who commit isolated sex offenses are not real sex deviates. They often have poorly organized egos and under noxious circumstances their defenses are momentarily broken down; alcohol or some personal catastrophe can do this. . . . Not infrequently a sexual offense may be the symptom of a psychosis. As a matter of fact nearly every variety of mental disorder may have this type of misconduct as a symptom. Characteristically, the senile arteriosclerotic becomes involved in pedophilia, the post encephalitic in impulsive aggressive attacks, the schizophrenic in unsolicited amorous advances both homosexual and heterosexual and the manic in exhibitionistic displays. But there is no constancy to this symptomatology.

Abrahamsen says there is no psychodynamic difference between sex offenders and other offenders, but sex offenders have been placed in a separate classification because of society's concern about the particular sex acts committed.†

A review of the historical development of society's attitudes about sex and sexual-offense legislation may clarify some of the difficulties involved in classification and management of the sex offender. Attitudes toward perversion have varied throughout history, from culture to culture and within cultures.

> The ancient Greeks practiced homosexuality and pedophilia with impunity. Mosaic Law, however, prohibits homosexuality and intercourse with animals, prescribing the death penalty for these offenses. The strongest religious sanction against these two sexual practices has been derived from the story of Sodom and Gomorrah, as given in the Book of Genesis, in the assumption that they were the sins for which their inhabitants were punished; hence the term "sodomy," which to this day is used to denote both.[1]

Krafft-Ebing and Kraepelin and other leading psychiatrists of the late nineteenth and early twentieth centuries considered sexual perversion to be essentially a form of "degeneracy" caused by a hereditary "taint" and often associated with physical stigmata of degeneracy. The United States Armed Forces Military Law considers that sexual misconduct does not in itself constitute a psychiatric category. Nevertheless, "command and court officials and the public in general, tend to lump all sex offenders into a single bracket and to consider them as 'degenerates,' 'maniacs,' etc."* As late as 1951 a judge in California, in a decision which unfortunately still stands, boldly expressed his archaic, in-

---

† Abrahamsen, "Governor's Report on the Study of 102 Sex Offenders of Sing Sing Prison" (1950) as cited in Guttmacher and Weihofen, *Psychiatry and the Law*, at 133. There is no distinct dividing line between sex offenders and other law violators . . . sex offenders have been found to suffer from no single category of mental pathology; the same varying symptoms of basic difficulties are also found in thieves, murderers, burglars and extortionists. Moreover, as police and probation records disclose, men who are primarily offenders often commit other types of crime and vice versa.

Sex offenders are in a separate classification only because of society's concern about their particular type of act, not because they differ widely from other criminals in the basic causes of their antisocial behavior.

* 8 *Psychiatry in Military Law* 240 (1953).

deed harmful, opinion on sex offenders. He denied the emotional component to sexual deviation and said that there is no treatment for these tendencies.†

It is obvious then that the attitudes of society, historically and traditionally, have been harsher and more punitive toward the sex offender than toward the general offender. Why has this been the case? What is it that society is attempting to control; the dangerous sexual offender or all sex offenders in general (or all sexual deviates)? The only sexual act with another person that is not a crime in most jurisdictions is coitus between married partners. The need to encourage propagation which gave rise to such harsh, rigid attitudes toward sexual activity has long since passed, but the attitude lingers on. It lingers on within each of us as individuals in our own sexual attitudes. The foreplay experienced and enjoyed in normal coitus is in part regressive behavior to earlier forms of "less mature" sexual functioning. As Karpman says, "Equally, there is something of the paraphiliac in everyone of us, and also something of the sexual psychopath."[1]

We react to our own sexual drives in many ways. Those that are acceptable, we express at the appropriate time and under the proper circumstances. The immature and socially unacceptable ones we must handle with the classical defenses of denial and repression. This would suffice if all people were successful in their defenses, but there are those who would dare to express these unacceptable and even possibly dangerous urges, thereby reminding us of our own drives which then need to be suppressed even further. Hence we institute social and community sanctions against such behavior to reinforce our own unconscious defense

---

† *People v. Hector,* 231 P.2d 916, 920 (1951) (dissenting opinion) . . . so far as the "treatment and rehabilitation" of these sexual perverts is concerned, there is no treatment and their "rehabilitation" is but a notion that exists only in the minds of fanatical social workers. . . .

Moreover, it is well known that these sexually abnormal acts are purely physical and in no sense mental. There has existed since the dawn of history, and history records brilliant mental achievements of men who were known to be victims of such offensive, obnoxious and repulsive sex abnormalities in some form or another. And there is no cure for these abnormalities or sexual tendencies, psychiatrists to the contrary notwithstanding.

mechanisms. The stronger the repressed drives are, the harsher need be the controls. In a larger sense, the answer lies within the mores of society, which are influenced by the individual mores, which in turn are products of development, education and parental moral values. That sexual mores of different jurisdictions vary is obvious, as reflected in the various penal codes. Sodomy, for example, is punishable by periods of confinement ranging from one to thirty years.*

Thus, it is felt that the confusion in our sexual offender laws reflects a general confusion of attitude toward sexual activity. Despite this confusion, science has made progressive inroads into the understanding of the sexual deviate. Freud's theory of the stages of sexual development, proposed in his *Three Contributions to the Theory of Sex* in 1905, has formed the basis of many current theories of neuroses and emotional disturbances. He postulates that a sexual perversion may arise either through arrest or fixation at an immature (pregenital) stage of development or through later return (regression) to that stage. The primal factor involved in perversion, according to Fenichel, is castration anxiety.† This factor is also primary in psychoneurosis.

Psychiatrists recognize that sex offenses and sexual deviation are related to general emotional and mental illness. Accordingly, all homosexuals, exhibitionists, voyeurs, transvestites, pedophiliacs, etc. are not suffering from the same mental aberration or personality disorder, but are individuals whose internal conflicts are resolved in a variety of ways, one of which is in an abnormal expression of sexual urges. The specificity of sexual deviation is significant in clarifying the misconception that "minor sex offenders" progress to major offenses. The latter can hardly be generally true, inasmuch as a particular expression of sexual gratification is utilized to resolve internal conflicts. Other sexual expressions would not aid in the resolution of such conflicts for that individual. For example, exhibitionists will often, under appropriate treatment, reveal the inadequate nature of heterosexual intercourse and the qualitatively different feeling they re-

* See *Cal Pen Code* §286 (not less than 1 yr); *Conn Gen Stat Ann* §53-216 (1960) (not more than 30 yr).
† Fenichel, *The Psychoanalytic Theory of Neurosis* 44 (1945).

ceive from masturbating and reaching an orgasm during an exhibitionistic act. In many cases, the gratification achieved is not solely for sexual pleasure, but for the resolution of internal conflicts involving feelings of adequacy as a man. For that individual, no such feeling of adequacy could be attained by forcible rape, for example, as it could by exhibitionistic orgasm.

On the other side of the coin, there are general nonsexual offenses, such as arson, kleptomania, burglary and murder, which have sexually motivating aspects. Breaking and entering or burglary by the adolescent is often equated with breaking and entering of the forbidden area of the female, as in rape. Even the term rape has the nonsexual meaning of pillaging and destroying. Contrary to popular notion, it is not the exhibitionist, but the burglar who is more likely to commit rape. This relationship is based not only on clinical observation and psychodynamic formulation, but also on criminal statistics.*

In summary, the following variations exist: all sex offenders are not sexually deviated; all sexual deviations do not become sexual offenses; some nonsexual offenses are motivated by sexual conflict; there are nonsexual conflicts that stimulate sexual deviation or offense; there are a variety of psychiatric conditions and dynamic factors which go into producing any one of the sexual offenses.

It becomes as ridiculous for the psychiatrist to label an individual an exhibitionist, a voyeur, a homosexual or a pedophiliac, as for the law to denote an exhibitionist as a sex offender or a sexual psychopath. An exhibitionist may be a mentally retarded individual or a schizophrenic, or he may be given other labels which are just as lacking in utility to the law as is the sexual psychopath appellation. As scientifically unsound as it is to lump all sex offenders into the same category, it is just as unreasonable to lump as "exhibitionists" all varieties of individuals who expose themselves or as "homosexuals" all males who engage in sexual relations with the same sex. Certainly, the individual is more complex than the single label attached, or even a double label, and should be presented in terms of a dynamic understanding

---

* Unpublished statistics from the files of the Philadelphia prison system.

of his behavior and not just a convenient over-simplified classification. It is helpful to the statistician, but not to the social scientist, nor to the judge, nor to the lawyer.

The law considers the individual merits of a case when it engages in the adversary procedure for the determination of guilt. The law has come to recognize that even all guilty rapists do not deserve the same sentence, and the law has requested consultation and dispositional recommendations from its advisers, the behavioral and social scientists (probation officers, court psychologists and psychiatrists). A presentence investigation has become an important and necessary aid to the judge and now has become the law of Pennsylvania for all individuals found guilty of crimes requiring a sentence of two years or more (unless the judge provides to the contrary).† In a presentence investigation, a thorough examination and appraisal of an individual's social, emotional and intellectual assets and liabilities is made. The judge is then in a position to impose an appropriate sentence for the offender and not for the offense.

In a similar manner psychiatrists are beginning to amplify their statements to the courts by elaborating on and clarifying the use of their labels. They do this by using dynamic formulations as well as behavioral predictions. This comprehensive forensic psychiatric reporting entails an understanding of the individual beyond the convenient labels that psychiatry has imposed for classification.

One of the important areas on the frontier of law and psychiatry with respect to the sexual offender, is the distinction between personal illness and danger to the community. A man may be both dangerous and personally ill; he may be either or neither. The law fails to distinguish between public nuisances and actual social menaces. Indecent exposure before children is a social menace; before adults it is only a nuisance.* Massachusetts attempted to improve its sexual offender laws in 1958 by changing the label of the "sexual psychopath" to the much more acceptable one (because dynamic rather than static) of "sexually

---

† *Pa Stat Ann* tit. 19, §890 (Supp. 1966).
* See Karpman, *The Sexual Offender and His Offenses* 460 (1954).

dangerous person." This confines the indeterminate sentence to those persons who show sexual aggression or violence and also to those who impose their sexual difficulties on individuals under the age of sixteen.†

These criteria are utilized for the indeterminate sentence only, and this law does not remove other nonaggressive sexual offenses from the general category of crime. However, the important consideration to be reviewed here is whether or not there ought to be a category of "sexual offenses" in the first place. This tends to be inaccurate and unrealistic and may be prejudicial to the male, in whom most of the sexual deviations exist. There are many instances in which a male is arrested for a serious sexual offense, and a female engaging in similar behavior would be either exculpated or indicted for a more minor offense.‡ In addition, the sexual motivation for many nonsexual offenses tends to dilute the significance of the term "sexual offense." Society has focused attention on the aggressive and sexual offenses primarily because our own acceptable urges are in the areas of sex and aggression. Recent statistics from the Forensic Psychiatry Clinic for the year 1965 to 1966 indicate that over half the referrals for psychiatric evaluation by the Defender Association of Philadelphia were for offenses involving sexual aggression. However, there are many offenses which involve nonaggressive sexual behavior, such as exhibitionism and voyeurism, which are recidivistic and annoying, but the individuals committing these acts are not necessarily dangerous, nor are they likely to become violent or dangerous individuals. Should these nonaggressive sexual offenses be classified with the aggressive ones?

It is suggested that for purposes of management, disposition, treatment and rehabilitation, the category of "sexual offenses" be dropped and no specialized legislation be passed to "handle the problem of the sex fiend." Individuals committing acts of violence and aggression, whether sexual or not, should be re-

---

† See Tenney, "Sex, Sanity and Stupidity in Massachusetts," 42 B.U.L. Rev. 1 (1962).

‡ For instance, there is no crime of assault with intent to rape for a woman, and indecent exposure is treated as a lesser offense than exhibitionism.

ferred for psychiatric evaluation to determine the potentiality for future violence or danger to the community, as well as the potentiality for future serious mental illness. Roughly 20 to 25 percent of the inmates at maximum security correctional institutions in Philadelphia are considered to be suffering from severe mental illness of psychotic or near-psychotic proportions.* These men must be identified as early as possible to give ample opportunity for treatment and rehabilitation and not merely incarcerated to remove them from society. Many of the most dangerous individuals are mentally ill or potentially so and must be given the opportunity for treatment.

This chapter has reviewed the psychiatric and legal labels given to the sexually deviated offender. It has been noted that there are inconsistencies among the legal definitions of the sexual psychopath and that there are various sexual deviations which do not fall within the criminal code. In addition there are crimes of an apparently nonsexual nature which do not stem from sexual deviation but rather from general antisocial tendencies. Adequate classification, both for the sex offender and for the sex deviation, is important in treating those in need and in using legal sanctions against those who menace the safety of the community.

The law must classify according to crime and behavior. A psychiatrist need not confine his diagnosis to labels alone. As an aid to the law and a consultant to the judge, the examining psychiatrist should provide a diagnostic formulation which transcends the labels imposed and which attempts to explain the offender as an individual, whether he be sexually deviated or not. With such an approach, each individual who comes before the law will be properly classified and evaluated so that he can be afforded treatment when necessary, and society may be protected as well. It is necessary that a cooperative effort among lawyers and psychiatrists be encouraged for appropriate classification of each individual offender. A plea is made to eliminate the prejudicial category of "sexual offender" or "sexual psychopath" as

---

* Unpublished statistics from the files of the Philadelphia prison system.

unscientific and emotionally charged labels, and to refer to so-called sexual offenders as individuals with a variety of problems that may be treated if properly evaluated and understood.

REFERENCES

1. Friedman, P.: Sexual deviations. In Arieti, S. (Ed.): *American Handbook of Psychiatry*, 589. New York, Basic Books, 1959.
2. Karpman, B.: The sexual psychopath. *J Crim LC & PS*, 42:184, 186, 1951.
3. Hacker, F. and Frym, M.: The sexual psychopath act in practice: A critical discussion. *Calif L Rev*, 43:766, 769-70, 1955.
4. Cleckley, H.: Psychopathic states. In Arieti, S. (Ed.): *American Handbook of Psychiatry*, 567, New York, Basic Books, 1959.

Chapter 13

ALCOHOL AND DRUGS

ONE OF THE MOST SIGNIFICANT problems psychiatrists and lawyers confront is the rising use and abuse of drugs and alcohol. Alcoholics have been shifted back and forth from management by the criminal justice system to treatment in the medical system. Drug addicts have medical problems but also run afoul of the law. Neither attorneys, judges, corrections officials nor physicians alone can handle the problem. Newer treatment methods have been devised which have shown some degree of success for drug addicts. Alcoholism continues on the rise and the AA programs have been shown to be most effective. Traditional medical treatment programs have not worked without added help from the law or from other nonmedical programs. A joint effort is required for the effective management and treatment of drug and alcohol abusers.

This chapter is not intended to pursue this problem in any great depth but rather to bring to the attention of both attorneys and psychiatrists some of the mutual difficulties we may encounter in dealing with individuals who have serious addiction problems.

On the civil side, a man who has been a chronic alcoholic for many years may be committed for treatment because he shows poor judgment and is considered a danger to himself. He may also present a problem of competency to manage his affairs if he has material substance. He may be declared incompetent so that he would not drink away his family's estate.

From the criminal point of view, the issues are much more clearly focused. Should the alcoholic or drug addict be treated as a criminal or as a medical problem? The decision has never been settled finally and these people have been bounced back and forth from one system to another in an attempt to provide optimal service. It becomes increasingly clear that neither system alone can manage the drug or alcohol abuser who is also involved in criminal matters. We need a combined approach; the alcoholic may be ill, but also may be criminal. Incarceration alone will not help his alcoholism; the medical treatment alone will not satisfy his rehabilitation for his criminal offense.

Lawyers must be familiar with the effects of alcohol and drugs upon a person. Generally there are five categories of drugs that are abused.

1. *Narcotics* are used primarily for the relief of pain and consist of morphine, heroin, Dilaudid® and Dolophine® (methadone).
2. *Barbiturates* are primarily used for sleep. They include amytal, pentothal, seconal, nembutal and tuinal. (They are often called "downers.")
3. *Amphetamines ("uppers")* are primarily used for narcolepsy or sleep disorders, also for weight control. They include Dexedrine®, Dexamyl® and Methedrine.®
4. *Psychedelics* including LSD, psilocybin and mescaline produce a psychotic-like state. Users speak of a "trip." Some may produce flashback phenomena years later when no drugs are being used.
5. *Tranquilizers** include Thorazine®, Stelazine®, Triavil®, Valium®, Librium®, Equanil®. The *Antidepressants* are Elavil®, Tofranil®, Marplan® and Parnate®. These drugs are used legitimately in psychiatric practice.

Perhaps a note here on the use of medication in psychiatry would be helpful to the practicing attorney. Drugs have always been used in the treatment of agitation and depression, but never as effectively as in the past twenty years. Pain has been relieved by use of cocaine or narcotics and bromides have helped to calm people's nerves. The most effective treatment until recently for depression was electroshock therapy. However, since

---

* Brand names are used in this chapter to identify the more commonly prescribed medications. Generic names would be confusing to the reader. No inferences should be drawn or assumptions made that these particular medications are superior or recommended. They are commonly prescribed for the ailments listed.

the phenothiazines *(Thorazine)* were found in 1954, to be effective for the treatment of schizophrenia, a number of different kinds of medication have been discovered and utilized in the treatment of psychotic illness, anxiety and depression. Many psychiatrists avoid the use of medication and prefer to use "talking therapy," rather than obtain a temporary relief of symptoms. However, the majority of psychiatrists do prescribe medication when appropriate.

Following is a general guideline to the nature of symptoms or illness for which specific kinds of medication are prescribed.

1. *Major mental illness or psychosis, schizophrenia,* with hallucinations or delusions: the major tranquilizers for the treatment of this type of psychosis are Thorazine, Mellaril®, Stelazine, Haldol®, Prolixin® and other major tranquilizers of a similar nature.
2. For the treatment of *severe depression,* Elavil, Tofranil, Pertofrane®, Marplan, Parnate and Marsilid have been found to be effective. In many cases where the medication is not effective, electroshock therapy remains a significant treatment choice.
3. For *manic illness* as a part of *manic depressive psychosis,* the specific medication has been found to be *lithium carbonate.*
4. *Anxiety* has been effectively managed by use of either major tranquilizers such as Stelazine or Mellaril, or the minor tranquilizers as Valium, Librium or meprobamate. Occasionally in a combination of anxiety and depression, psychiatrists have found combined medications such as Triavil (Trilafon and Elavil) to be effective. Others will combine two different kinds of drugs such as Stelazine and Elavil so they may regulate the dosage of each. Mellaril, Stelazine or Valium may be useful in calming anxiety and reduce depressive feelings stimulated by the anxiety.

Recently a number of other newer medications have come on the market. For a detailed description of any type of medication prescribed, with its side effects, contraindications and toxic effect, the reader is referred to the Physician's Desk Reference

(PDR)[1] which is published yearly by *Medical Economics*. Physicians consult this manual for optimal prescribing dosages and for cautionary notices for themselves and for alerting patients.

Alcohol remains the most widely abused drug and is considered to be a depressant rather than a stimulant. People may become "high" or stimulated initially, but the major effect is one of depression.

The question arises as to what constitutes an "alcoholic" or an "addict." Many drugs will cause habituation; i.e. the person will continue to utilize the drug because he finds it to be a pleasant habit. One is considered to be physically addicted only when there is a physiological reaction to withdrawing the medication. The body develops a tolerance to the drug by requiring greater amounts with each usage. It is not unknown, for example, for people who have become habituated with amphetamines to be able to take from eighty to one hundred, 10 mgm tablets a day without significant effect. Others who are not addicted or habituated may take one or two, 10 mgm tablets and feel high for many hours.

The addicting drugs are primarily the narcotics, including heroin and morphine; heavy users will show physical withdrawal symptoms lasting between twenty-four to seventy-two hours at peak. Occasionally the person withdrawing does not feel well until about one hundred or more hours have passed. The primary symptoms are abdominal cramps, nasal discharge, a feeling of malaise, diarrhea, vomiting and anorexia. Often the person withdrawing from narcotics will feel better and withdraw more readily if he is certain that he will not receive any medication for his withdrawal symptoms.

Withdrawing from barbiturates may be a different story, since withdrawal may result in convulsions which could lead to death. A barbiturate addict should never withdraw outside of a hospital and without proper medical care. An amphetamine addict may show signs of serious depression and suicide on withdrawal from his medication. There is no addiction to the psychedelics or marijuana. There is occasionally addiction to alcohol resulting in delirium tremens (D.T.'s).

Many people have discussed the definition of an alcoholic. Some have said if a person has to drink every day or if he cannot function without alcohol, he is an alcoholic. Others have placed the emphasis on functioning effectively; i.e. if a person misses work because of alcohol intake, he is an alcoholic. The author's definition is that if a person needs to finish the bottle, or drink until he is unconscious or sick, then he is an alcoholic. This is implied by the fact that he has such an overwhelming urge to continue drinking that he has no internal control over his behavior. External controls such as a state of unconsciousness, gastric upset with vomiting or absence of alcohol will cause the alcoholic to stop drinking at that time. The true addict does not save half the bottle for tomorrow. For him, there is no tomorrow.

This presentation is not a detailed treatise on the medical or social effects of alcohol or drug abuse. For a more detailed treatment of these problems the reader is referred to standard textbooks on alcoholism and drug abuse. Ungerleider's treatise of *The Problems and Prospects of LSD*,[2] *Marijuana Reconsidered*, by Grinspoon[3] and other good references, as is David Musto's book, *The American Disease*.[4] Dr. Musto describes the origins of narcotics control and discusses the history of drug abuse in America.

For the forensic psychiatrist or lawyer involved in criminal matters the following two notes apply. The first deals with the concept of flashback phenomena following LSD "trips." In a number of people the author has examined, it was found that excessive alcohol intake may stimulate a flashback phenomenon in which the individual may react with hallucinations, delusions and related violent behavior, even homicide. In one case, a young man who had killed another person claimed that he had not remembered. Others insisted that he "becomes crazy" when he drinks. To test this phenomena alcohol in a controlled test dose (95% ethyl alcohol mixed in a 3-1 solution with fruit juice) was administered. After 63 cc of alcohol were ingested, the patient noted visual distortions characteristic of LSD intake but not characteristic of alcohol intoxication. After 125 cc of alcohol were ingested, the patient became psychotic, violent and uncontrollable. He had a subsequent amnesia for this period of time which was ultimately controlled by Thorazine injection.

In the second case the individual had discontinued LSD usage after a frightening experience under its effect. He drank more heavily and noted increasing visual and auditory hallucinations. One day at work, in a paranoid deluded state, he killed his co-worker by repeated knife stabs.

It is the author's impression that in both cases alcohol served as a stimulating effect to the psychotic condition often referred to as "flashback" following LSD ingestion. Since these two cases communication with others corroborates this impression and two other cases with similar relationships have been witnessed.

The second note is contained in a paper published in the *Bulletin* of the American Academy of Psychiatry and the Law (formerly the Newsletter of AAPL) by Dr. Bruce Danto and the author.[5] Dr. Danto had examined an individual in a prison who claimed that he was under the influence of LSD when he committed the crime, and pleaded insanity. Dr. Danto found on careful examination that the individual had been deceptive and had not used LSD at all. He was making up the symptoms after he had spoken with others in the prison, but had confused the appearance of LSD and its effects on him.

By contrast, the author had examined an individual who had demonstrated true LSD intoxication while he committed a bank robbery. He did not immediately come up with a "story" that he was on LSD, but was confused even at the police station. It was later determined that he was indeed a heroin addict and had been on LSD that morning. He had a partial amnesia lasting several hours. In contrast to Dr. Danto's case, this man had not planned the project with anyone else or in as careful detail as was obvious in the first case. He acted spontaneously and in response to erratic stimuli.

These cases illustrate the caution with which the forensic psychiatrist and attorney should approach voluntary statements regarding insanity pleas while under the influence of LSD. Careful questioning regarding specifics and details of the state of intoxication will prove whether or not they are consistent with known clinical experiences. Attorneys interviewing clients claiming drug intoxication at the time of crime or during confession should obtain psychiatric examination and consultation.

Proper evaluation of drug and alcohol problems is essential in criminal matters. Treatment of alcoholics and addicts remains a medical problem but often requires community, family and legal help.

REFERENCES

1. *Physician's Desk Reference*. 28th ed. Oradell, Medical Economics, 1974.
2. Ungerleider, T.: *The Problems and Prospects of LSD*. Springfield, Thomas, 1968.
3. Grinspoon, L.: *Marijuana Reconsidered*. Cambridge, Harvard U Pr, 1971.
4. Musto, D.: *The American Disease*. New Haven, Yale U Pr, 1973.
5. Danto, B. and Sadoff, R. L.: LSD and the insanity plea: A note of caution. *Newsletter*, AAPL, Vol II, #2, Jan., 1971.

SECTION III

THE PSYCHIATRIST AND CIVIL LAW

THIS SECTION CONSISTS of five chapters primarily devoted to the practical role of the psychiatrist in various aspects of civil law. Traditionally psychiatrists have been called upon to examine individuals involved in civil-legal difficulties in these areas:

A. Family and domestic relations, including conflicts and problems of marriage, divorce, annulment, child custody and visitation privileges
B. Actions in tort involving traumatic neuroses or psychoses, emotional conditions following trauma, workmen's compensation and cases of negligence and malpractice
C. Commitment procedures, both voluntary and involuntary
D. Competency determinations including competency to manage one's own affairs, guardianship procedures, testamentary capacity, competency to run a business, to vote, to get married, to be a witness, to drive, etc.

Some of the newer procedures in which psychiatric testimony is utilized more frequently, illustrating the expanding role of psychiatry in civil law, are the following:

A. An increase and change in the number and kinds of evaluations for therapeutic abortion
B. Greatly expanded use of psychiatric evaluation and treatment for drug abuse cases
C. Psychiatric testimony in committed patients with a right to adequate treatment in hospital
D. Psychiatric examination of victims of crimes; for example, victims of sex offenses
E. Comprehensive exploration of family dynamics with the hope of preventing family disruption

F. Increased and expanded use of psychiatric testimony in workmen's compensation cases

The general psychiatrist will more than likely be exposed to the problems involved in commitments and in domestic relations matters rather than criminal matters. He may also become involved in evaluating people who have been injured, with subsequent emotional sequellae.

This section covers the basic functions of the forensic psychiatrist in the civil matters outlined. It does not delve into the newer procedures listed in this introduction. Again, this section is a practical guide for attorneys and psychiatrists working together in the increasing complexity of civil-legal forensic psychiatry.

Chapter 14

PSYCHIATRIC ASSESSMENT OF MENTAL COMPETENCY

PERHAPS THE MOST IMPORTANT area in forensic psychiatry for the psychiatrist to understand is that of competency. Competency is an all-encompassing term which has specific meaning as a legal word of art. Generally when we speak of competency we may be referring to a person's ability to handle his own affairs, and whether or not he needs a guardian appointed. This is certainly one important type of competency and one in which the psychiatrist often is called for his opinion.

In many states this type of incompetency is automatic with commitment procedures; i.e. when a patient is committed to a hospital he is also declared incompetent and a guardian is appointed. Thus, the individual is not able to vote, to own property, to sue in court or to pursue other aspects of his civil rights as a competent citizen.

However, in most states competency is not automatically connected with commitment. One may be committed to a state hospital and maintain his civil rights and not be considered legally incompetent.

Generally speaking, for a person to be declared incompetent he lacks the ability to know the extent of his material holdings or to handle his affairs wisely and prudently. A man need not be psychotic to be incompetent; he may be a spendthrift, or an alcoholic, or in some way be unable to control the spending of his money, or be readily subject to the influence of designing persons. Basically the test for competency is designed to keep the family from losing its wealth and/or properties.

If an individual is evaluated for competency he should certainly be aware of the extent of his bounty, use relatively good judgment and be able to add and subtract. Mental retardation in this respect would be appropriate for declaration of incompetency in many cases, as would drug addiction, alcoholism, compulsive gambling, psychosis and "one who is excessively easily led." It should be remembered that in a declaration of incompetency for general affairs, as in any other declaration of incompetency, it is the court and not the psychiatrist who makes such a declaration. The psychiatrist merely acts as a consultant to the court as he does in all other instances in forensic psychiatry.

The author usually teaches students not to answer the question, "What is competency?" by a direct statement, but to utilize the time honored psychiatric ploy of responding with another question: "Competency to do what?" This is essential because specific medical-legal criteria for competency differs, according to the specific needs of the declaration. For example, testamentary capacity, the mental capacity to prepare a will, is much different from the mental capacity required to marry, or to stand trial or even to be executed.

Testamentary Capacity

In order for a person to prepare a valid will, he must have the following criteria of mental competency or testamentary capacity: (1) to know that he is making a will; (2) the nature and extent of his bounty; (3) the existence of his heirs and their relationship to him. He need not leave his money to his heirs; he may be psychotic, an alcoholic or a spendthrift or a compulsive gambler and still be competent to prepare a will if he knows he is making a will, how much money he has and who are the natural objects of his bounty and affection.

However, there is another aspect of testamentary capacity which is not usually spelled out by these criteria; i.e. a will may be declared invalid if it can be proven that at the time of the signing of the will the testator was suffering from such a state of mind that he was unduly influenced by conniving individuals.

An example of such a case may be an old man in a hospital, under the influence of medication,, surrounded by well-meaning relatives who influence him to change his will while he is in a state of complete dependency, anxiety and confusion. He may still know that he is making a will, how much money he has and who his relatives are, but he may be unduly influenced at the time, thus establishing a question of validity of the will. All this, of course, needs to be proven in a court of law under proper legal procedures in the usual adversary system.

Competency to Marry and Divorce

In order for a person to be competent to marry, he must know that he is getting married and must know the consequences of his vows. If he is in a stupor, or a state of confusion, and doesn't know that a ceremony is taking place, the marriage may be annulled on the basis of his incompetency. Other factors leading to annulment of a marriage may be fraud or deception of a prior illness or sterility; a bad reputation on the part of an older woman marrying a juvenile or young man; or withholding information such as the spouse not willing to have children, while indicating before the marriage that he was so willing.

Competency to be divorced is an interesting and often difficult concept to grasp. In any legal proceeding the rule stands that an individual must be both physically and mentally present. A divorce hearing, after all, is a contest where one person is blaming the other for doing something wrong in the marriage. Divorce may not proceed, e.g. in Pennsylvania (and in some other states) where the defendant spouse is in a mental hospital unless testimony can prove he is suffering from an "incurable mental illness" or has been hospitalized for a specific number of years. This rule was established primarily to protect mentally ill wives from being abandoned financially, and becoming destitute if or when her illness cleared.

Competency and Contracts

Competency to enter into a contract or business, or to sue, may be lumped into one general category: a person is competent in these matters only if he understands the nature of the proceeding in which he is involving himself; i.e. he must understand the nature of the business deal to prevent fraudulent practices against an unwitting individual. If it is proven that at the time of entering into an agreement or contract or a business deal, one partner was so incompetent that he did not understand or know the nature of the proceedings in which he was involving himself, then the contract may be declared null and void. It is usually required that a psychiatrist examine the individual and testify as to his mental state at the time of entering into the contract.

Different degrees of competency may exist in the same individual for various purposes, e.g. when one may be competent to vote but not to drive. The difference occasionally is confusing when the examination is of an elderly person for competency to manage his own affairs. The following case will illustrate the disparity in competency to manage one's own affairs and to prepare a will.

> An eighty-six-year-old woman was recently examined at a nursing home and it was found that she was incompetent to manage her affairs and was in need of a guardian. She did not know or understand the intricacies of managing her money or exactly how much she had in what form. The author was asked to examine her primarily because of a legal contest between her son and grandchildren about the management of her estate and the ultimate distribution of her wealth. Despite the fact that she could not manage her affairs and was aware that she could not, she knew generally how much money she had, who were the natural objects of her affection and to whom she could leave her money if she chose.
>
> Thus she had, in my opinion, testamentary capacity i.e. competency to write a will, but was in need of a guardian to manage her affairs.

Competency Evaluation to Aid Attorney

One interesting aspect of competency is that of evaluation of a client in order to aid the attorney in proceeding with his case. The client may be an individual who appears bizarre or unusual and makes strange accusations against someone else who is "out to get him." It is essential for the attorney to be certain of the mental status of his client before he proceeds to investigate the content of the charges brought by the client; i.e. is the client paranoid? Is he suffering from delusions that have no basis in reality? A clear example of this type of individual is represented by the following case.

A forty-one-year-old married, black woman was referred for evaluation of her complaint about a "plot" to disfigure her ten children. She complained of her husband's mother as being a "witch" from South Carolina who had powers to destroy her and her children. She related a fantastic tale of poison sumac being rubbed into the skin and over the eye of her ten-year-old child, causing the child to become blind in that eye. She was in the process of divorcing her husband and felt that her husband's mother, who was against the divorce, was retaliating by disfiguring her children.

Her attorney properly became suspicious of her mental status because of the bizarreness of her story, and referred her for psychiatric evaluation prior to proceeding with her complaint. Since her veracity was challenged, she brought with her to the interview neighbors who appeared to be reliable and corroborated her story. She was encouraged to write down the details of her difficulties and perhaps to try and get evidence for such a "plot." She seemed encouraged that someone had believed her yet she did not return for further evaluation, nor did she return for further legal advice.

This case reflects the difficulties noted in requesting psychiatric consultation; i.e. clients often become offended and discouraged from proceeding further with their claims.

One case of determination of competency brought to light a difficult situation in which an eighty-year-old man was under guardianship to his son because of his prior declaration of incompetency. The patient's wife had urged her attorney to attempt to have the guardianship removed on the basis of restoration of competency because of rehabilitative efforts following several strokes. The family was against such release of guardianship and protested. Psychiatric evaluation indicated that the "incompetent" had chronic brain syndrome, following a cerebral vascular accident with residual aphasia and memory loss. He was not psychotic and showed no evidence for hallucinations or delusions, but remained incompetent to manage his own affairs in that he was unable to show satisfactory memory or good judgment. The difficulty was not in the determination of his mental state, but in managing the problems he was having with his guardian, who was allowing him a less than adequate sum on which to live. His guardian happened to be his son and heir, who wished to maintain the estate intact, rather than to allow his ward to utilize the funds during his lifetime. The situation was brought to light at a hearing and produced an increase in the allotment of funds to the incompetent individual by his guardian, satisfying the patient and his wife.

One final case illustrates the difference between the substantive criteria for competency and subjection to undue influence.

The author was asked to examine a seventy-year-old black, widowed, retired railroad engineer by the attorney for his daughter, with whom he was living. The house was owned by father and daughter jointly. She also had two married sisters who had taken little responsibility for their father except during the recent year. He had become increasingly blind and hard-of-hearing. He had also developed a condition of his colon which required surgery and follow-up medical care with adequate diet. The sister who had been caring for her father noted that during this period of hospitalization her two other sisters had visited him in the hospital and influenced him to withdraw his money from his bank account and put it into a bank nearer to them, with one of the sisters as cosigner. The question became a family problem about who would manage the funds and utilize them.

It was shown that the funds had been withdrawn in order to pay expenses for the other sister's family. In this case the author made a house call and examined the old man, who was cooperative and willing to talk. He seemed a bit defensive but was able to understand the nature of my visit and did know how much money he had, where it was and how it was to be handled. He did not appear to be incompetent from the standpoint. However, it was shown that he needed care and that he was overly dependent on others for his physical and medical condition. Without the help of a housekeeper, he would deteriorate physically and would not attend to his medical requirements. From a purely medical point of view, this man required care and attention. From a psychiatric point of view, he was not incompetent to manage his own affairs but was subject to the will of other persons (designing, conniving).

At the hearing all parties involved recognized his dependent state and recommended a guardian be appointed. The issue was not his competency but rather, who would control the funds and act as guardian.

This case is presented primarily to distinguish classical criteria for mental competency, as opposed to dependency with need for care to prevent undue influence. In this instance the psychiatrist acts as a physician as well as a specialist in mental problems in assessing the patient's overall needs and medical requirements.

Competency in Criminal Proceedings

There are many areas in the criminal process wherein the individual, or defendant, may be declared incompetent to proceed. At the beginning the suspect being interrogated may be incompetent to make a confession or to waive various rights: to remain silent, to obtain legal counsel, to a jury. He may be mentally retarded to the point of not understanding the questions presented to him by the interrogating officers. He may be so deluded or psychotic at the time that a confession for him was his means of salvation from problems worse than jail (e.g. a drug addict experiencing withdrawal). He may be found incompetent to proceed at any level of the criminal procedure, including preliminary hearing and arraignment.

The most important area of competency in criminal law is competency to stand trial. Criteria for this determination are the following: he must know the nature of the proceedings in which he is involved; he must be able to work with counsel in preparing a rational defense; he must be of sufficient mental stability that the stress of trial will not precipitate a deterioration in his condition to a psychotic state. These factors often are quite easy to determine, but in many cases could be very difficult, especially whether or not the defendant is able to confer with counsel in preparing a rational defense.

This aspect may be more difficult to determine when the defendant is not allowed to speak to the examining psychiatrist about his crime. In some instances competency at time of trial may have to be determined only at the time the trial occurs.

Other areas of competency include (1) to proceed to be sentenced. (Is he competent to spend time in jail or will that cause further deterioration of his condition? Will he need a hospital instead?) (2) to be executed. (This appears to be based on humanitarian reason, but also on the notion that if a person is *non compis mentis*, that is, not competent to be executed, he should not be, because if he were competent he may come up with that bit of information which could save his life.) (3) To be placed on probation or parole.

In summary, it is important for the student of forensic psychiatry to note the various types of competency in which he may be called upon to evaluate an individual. He should always ask for what purpose the competency evaluation is occurring, and evaluate the patient for specific medical-legal criteria, in addition to the general psychiatric examination.

Chapter 15

PSYCHIATRIC CONSULTATION IN DOMESTIC RELATIONS MATTERS

DOMESTIC RELATIONS CASES raise many challenges to the consulting psychiatrist. Divorce is usually a private legal matter in which psychiatrists may be called for consultation primarily to examine one or both parties. Often the consultation is requested to be certain that the parties to the divorce understand what their situation involves, especially where children are concerned. Occasionally it is a matter of marriage counseling to aid the disputing parties. Proceedings for child custody and visitation rights often raise problems requiring court appointed psychiatric consultation, as well as private psychiatric evaluation. It is especially helpful when families involved in such matters are referred by the judge for evaluation, since in that situation all parties must appear for examination by order of the court. It is essential that all family members be examined and evaluated in the determination of such an important decision.

Ordinarily in such domestic relations matters the psychiatrist is called by one side or the other and is able to see only one parent, usually the one raising the legal challenge.

In one fairly tragic case, an eleven-year-old boy was given in custody to his mother by court order. Mother moved away from Pennsylvania to New York and lived in a rather poor, ill-kept home on the beach. The boy complained to his father, who had visitation rights every other weekend, that he was not being properly cared for. He said he was punished by mother's boyfriend and deprived of friends of his own. He said he hated to return and always presented an emotional reaction at the time he was to return to New York after visiting for the weekend with his father in upstate Pennsylvania.

After several such weekends, with increasing depression on the part of his son, the father decided to keep the son in Pennsylvania and risk legal action by his former wife. Indeed, the boy's mother did bring an action against the father for keeping the child against the court order granting custody to the mother. A psychiatrist from New York presented expert psychiatric testimony that the boy was better off with his mother, that she was a better parent to him than was the father. The author testified that the father was an adequate father, a good father, but there was no way that a comparison with the boy's mother could be made because no examination of her or the relationship between the boy and his mother had been made. The author commented that he did not understand how the psychiatrist from New York would be able to make such a comparison without having the opportunity to examine and interview the father.

The judge recognized the limitation on our testimony and subsequently ordered a neutral psychiatrist to examine all parties in the matter before rendering a decision. Such action by courts in order to prevent the kind of biased testimony not based on comprehensive and complete examination that so often occurs in domestic relations matters is advisable.

Psychiatric examination is hampered by a limited evaluation and presents only a partial picture of the overall situation. Ideally, families referred by judges allow for a more comprehensive evaluation and the psychiatrist may function as a true consultant to the court, unhampered by an adversary position. Two cases will illustrate this distinction.

Case Number One

In the first instance, the psychiatrist was called as a consultant by a private attorney representing a mother who had custody of three children and was concerned that the visitation by her ex-husband, the father of the children, was damaging to their emotional condition. The children were examined individually and together, and each in the presence of their mother. The mother was seen individually and complained that her ex-husband had been diagnosed by another psychiatrist as a paranoid schizophrenic; she also detailed his behavior, which seemed to be quite unusual and bizarre, and certainly resembled the behavior of a psychotic individual. The husband, of course, was not willing to submit to a psychiatric examination since he felt it was not warranted and did not feel that his mental state should be questioned.

The children did not wish to see their father and felt that he was cruel, since he had broken into the house during one holiday period and had threatened and harmed their mother. They had been afraid of him and his impulsive outbursts and showed symptoms of emotional disturbance following each visitation. The mother was afraid that her ex-husband would abscond with the children to another part of the United States without her permission. It would be a simple matter for an adversary psychiatrist to state categorically that the presence of the father was emotionally damaging to the mental health of the children. He could then recommend no further visitations. However, he had not had a chance to examine the father and could not be certain that all accusations against the father were valid. Thus a compromise situation was worked out that the children would be visited in the presence of a mutually trusted friend for brief duration and limited frequency.

Case Number Two

The complaining mother charged that her ex-husband was mentally ill and cruel to their five-year-old daughter and that his visitation ought to be discontinued. The child was seen initially with her mother and she appeared to be quite sad, depressed and withdrawn. She stated that she did not wish to see her father, that he was cruel and mean to her. The mother supported these contentions and indicated that after each visitation the child exhibited nightmares, bedwetting and emotional regression. On examination, the father seemed to be a fairly reasonable, though nervous, individual who was claiming similar destructive effect on his daughter by his ex-wife. In the presence of her father the child became quite frightened and cool toward him. Because psychiatric evaluation was conducted and he was deemed not dangerous nor likely to harm the child, another compromise visitation was arranged whereby the father would see his daughter for two months during the summer and on holidays without the disruption that often occurs with weekly visits. On examination of the child alone and with her father, following the two-month summer reunion, she seemed much more cheerful, alert, less depressed and much warmer to her father, whom she had learned to love when not in the presence of her mother.

As in most difficult decisions involving human relations, compromise is often necessary. In both cases outlined, compromise was utilized, but in the latter case it was much more logically determined with greater confidence on the part of the psychiatric consultant. It is essential in domestic relations cases, wherever possible, that all parties involved be examined both alone and in concert, since often the individual factors are not the determining ones but rather, the dynamic interrelationship between and among members of the disrupted family.

In addition to the classic examination of parents and children for child custody determinations or visitation rights, a most significant aspect of such consultation involves the examination of family problems in which one spouse complains about the sanity of the other. This is especially important when the complained-of spouse is unwilling to appear for psychiatric examination.

These cases are especially difficult for the referring attorneys because in most instances the complained-of spouse would not appear for examination. In one case the spouse did appear with the following result.

> A thirty-five-year-old black female requested help from the Legal Aid Society because she was afraid her husband was going to kill her. He had threatened to do so and had attempted it once prior to his hospitalization. At that time, during an argument, she was cut with a knife, following which she called the police and had her husband taken to jail and then to the hospital. Upon his discharge from the hospital, he re-

turned home without informing his wife specifically when he would be home. She claims he had threatened to kill her again with a knife and she had left home because she was afraid of him and did not wish to chance his mental state. At the time of the interview she was hiding from him, pending a divorce that she had sought.

Examination of the husband indicated that he was a forty-year-old black male who couldn't understand why his wife had left home since he claimed he did not threaten her, nor did he attempt to harm her since his release from the hospital. He admitted he was nervous and upset, and could not sleep, but did not fight with her.

He described the marital situation as deteriorating for the previous two years, when she came home drunk after being at an all-night party without him, and he scolded her for her behavior. Since that time they had slept in separate bedrooms and had not had marital relations. He explained the fight in which he cut her as a culmination of marital tension that had built up over the previous two years, but stated that he did not wish to kill her, nor did he intend to harm her. He stated he would take her back under the following conditions: (1) that they sleep in the same room, though not necessarily demanding sexual relations; (2) that she keep the house in proper order; (3) that the children be well cared for; (4) that they attend church regularly with him and (5) that she behave like a lady.

It became obvious after talking with the complained-of spouse that he was not severely mentally ill, nor in need of psychiatric treatment. It was apparent that this was a marital discord in which both parties seemed to have difficulties. It was helpful indeed from the standpoint of the referring attorney, to have the report on the spouse, indicating that he had some compulsive difficulties, with obsessions and ruminations, and that he appeared to be frightening because of his authoritarian commanding manner, mixed with histrionic and dramatic gesturing. However, he did not appear to be dangerous, nor was there any fear that he would lose control of himself. It was determined that this was a marital problem in need of counseling. The extensive psychiatric evaluation provided the attorney with a clearer picture of the overall situation.

A similar case represents the value of a *joint interview:*

A forty-eight-year-old white woman also complained about her husband's history of mental hospitalization and his threat to abuse and harm her. It was felt that a joint interview would be helpful in determining the difficulties involved. In this case the husband appeared with his wife and was extremely defensive at the beginning, wishing to know why he was being interviewed. Following his initial defensive reaction, he became quite talkative and discussed most of the difficulties that he was having in relation to his wife's nagging. He presented as a fairly compulsive, rigid individual, who had many needs which were unrealistic, especially with regard to his wife's and children's attitudes.

It was determined from the joint interview that the problem in the family was one between both parents and certainly all the blame could not be placed on either party alone. During the interview it was revealed that the husband admitted that he became very depressed in the past and had been quite withdrawn, and may have aggravated the family difficulties. Both were willing to undergo psychiatric treatment because both felt it would be helpful to them, not only in their family situation, but also to them personally. The initial complaint by the wife was to have her husband committed to the state hospital because she felt he was dangerous. Following the psychiatric evaluation it was determined that he was not dangerous and that she was manipulating the situation to get him evaluated. As it occurred, they followed through with the recommendations for treatment and began work on their personal and family difficulties.

Following is a case wherein the complained-of spouse refused to be evaluated, raising the need for emergency community action for involuntary psychiatric examination and commitment:

Mrs. S, a twenty-nine-year-old married, black, female was re-referred for evaluation of her husband's mental state. She was concerned about her safety and the safety of her eight children because of her husband's threats to kill them. He had threatened to kill the children—the baby first—if she had ever left the house. His screaming and threatening became a repeated event, culminating in her decision to take the children from the house. In addition to the threats, she described him as mentally disturbed for the following reasons: he had hit her "every night for the past few months," and told her stories which sounded like fantasy; i.e. that he had a child before they were married and both the mother and the child had died. Later he said that these people did not exist and he had told her this because the "voice" came to him and told him to tell her. Furthermore, he felt he was chosen to "lead the Negro people" and he felt he was "special."

It seemed likely, based on description offered by Mrs. S, that her husband was suffering from an acute paranoid psychotic reaction, but this diagnosis would need to be corroborated and confirmed by direct examination. Since Mr. S was unwilling voluntarily to appear for evaluation, it was recommended that he be examined by mental health authorities with reference to involuntary commitment. Appropriate medical-legal action was taken; Mr. S was evaluated and found to be psychotic, dangerous to his wife and family and he was involuntarily committed to the state mental hospital, where he received intensive treatment.

One might question the active intervention of mental health authorities as a breach of Mr. S's civil rights; nevertheless, it was determined to be an emergency situation requiring immediate community-coordinated efforts to prevent a tragedy to the family. The evidence for such action was deemed significant and sufficient.

No-fault Divorce

As the number of states passing no-fault divorce laws increases, psychiatric consultation for evaluation and marriage counseling is also on the rise. Many of the statutes provide for mandatory or voluntary counseling, especially where children are involved. Often the provision is for counseling at the end of a waiting period consistent with the regulation for living apart before the final termination of marriage occurs. We have encouraged legislatures to provide for voluntary rather than mandatory marriage counseling and also to provide this counseling at the beginning of the waiting period, rather than at the end, when little or no benefit will be gained.

A number of lawyers have requested further information and training in family law and psychiatric concepts of marital psychodynamics and family interaction. Mostly, attorneys are concerned about doing the proper job as an attorney when a person comes to them with questions about marriage or divorce. However, they are also concerned about not giving advice which would be incompatible with good mental health recommendations. In a course, "Practical Applications of Family Law," offered to practicing attorneys in Philadelphia at the Marriage Council of Philadelphia (University of Pennsylvania) we had stressed interview techniques, underlying concerns of clients who request divorce proceedings and primarily when to refer for marriage counseling or psychiatric consultation.

Most attorneys are concerned about the general welfare of their clients, rather than merely getting the divorce when asked. Mostly they recognize that people seeking divorce have emotional problems attendant with their marital disruption and have become sensitive to their role as counselors as well as attorneys. Some prefer to maintain a purely legal role with their clients while others prefer to serve a mental health function in counseling their clients as well. We have recommended a middle course, in which the attorney considers his role as lawyer a priority while recognizing and dealing with underlying and attendant emotional difficulties.

We have also counseled psychiatrists and marriage counselors in dealing with legal problems encountered in their clients and patients. A very helpful presentation is made by Whitaker and Miller when they write,

We believe that psychiatric intervention when divorce impends cannot be regarded as a routine matter. The therapist should view his entrance into the situation as calling for his broadest perspective. He must see what is going on between him and his patient, already a difficult task. Even more than that, he must see what is implied by the fact that he and his patient are sitting down together without the mate. Any move by the therapist that discounts the significance of the marriage may be unexpectedly influential. Thus, the ordinary medical system or replying affirmatively to a request for help by one person in a marriage, excluding the other, may in effect be an intervention favoring divorce.[1]

They conclude with a statement which applies not only to psychiatrists but to consulting attorneys as well. "An observation passed down through the generations advises that almost any couple during a lifetime of marriage could find ample opportunity to break up, depending upon who is around when divorce impends. We hope that it will not be one of us." This is not to indicate that a lawyer should not be helpful to people who legitimately want and require a divorce; it is meant, however, to be a cautionary statement that we are sensitive to and aware of the ramifications and consequences of divorce in our society.

Briscoe and others from St. Louis found that, "three fourths of our divorced women and two thirds of our divorced men had, or currently have, a psychiatric illness. . . . Primary unipolar affective disease (depression) and antisocial personality in both men and women and hysteria in women, occurred more frequently in the divorce sample than in the control."[2] That is to say, the finding by Briscoe and his co-workers show that psychiatric illness occurred more frequently in divorced men and women than in nondivorced people. They are not saying whether the illness is caused by the divorce or concomitant with it.

Often it is quite helpful in domestic relations matters for the psychiatrist and attorney to work closely together. It is especially important in this matter. There may be legal questions the patient raises with the psychiatrist that he cannot answer and needs to discuss with the attorney. Similarly, the client will bring personal problems into the lawyer's consultation room with which he may feel uncomfortable and should feel free to relay these matters to the psychiatrist.

Especially in domestic relations matters it is important for the attorney to be aware of transference phenomena; i.e. the feelings of his client depending upon him in a very difficult and sensitive social matter as divorce. The dependent woman will rely heavily upon her attorney and those with hysterical features may be very seductive in attempting to obtain as much help as possible. The attorney must be sensitive to the client's needs and to unrealistic demands that might be made, especially when attorney and client are of the opposite sex.

REFERENCES

1. Whittaker, C. A., and Miller, M. H.: A re-evaluation of psychiatric help when divorce impends. *Am J Psychiat, 126*:5, 1969.
2. Briscoe, C. W., Smith. J. B., Robins, E., Martin, S., and Gaskin, F.: Divorce and psychiatric disease. *Arch Gen Psychiat, 29*, 1973.

Chapter 16

A PSYCHIATRIC VIEW OF INSANITY IN ANNULMENT AND DIVORCE

TERMINATION OF A MARRIAGE in which one partner is insane has produced a number of legal and medical-legal difficulties in the development of Domestic Relations Law. First, insanity may be a basis for annulment if the disorder existed at the time the marriage began.* Secondly, postnuptial onset of insanity may be presented either as grounds for divorce in some jurisdictions or as a defense to divorce on grounds other than insanity.[1]

Much of the difficulty that has arisen can be attributed to the various interpretations of the word "insanity" as viewed in each of these procedures. There are varying degrees or definitions of insanity depending on what legal procedure is considered.

A recent study conducted by the American Bar Foundation reveals the following situation in the various jurisdictions. "There is no uniformity in the language of the statutes which prohibits marriage of the mentally disabled. The list of terms describing the person affected by these laws is almost endless. Among the most common of these terms are idiots, insane, weak-minded lunatics, feeble-minded, imbeciles, persons incapable of contracting, and persons of unsound mind."[1] The study concludes, "It is still difficult to determine to whom the statutes apply and whether their scope is related to medical knowledge."[1]

The situation is even more complex when insanity is presented as a grounds for divorce or as a defense to divorce on other grounds. Distinctions have been made in the courts between the

---

First published in *Penna Bar Ass'n Q*, Vol. 37, Mar. 1966. Reprinted with permission.

* "At common-law a marriage with a lunatic was not merely voidable but void." *Hoadley v. Hoadley* 244, N.Y. 424, 155 NE 728 (1927).

degree of insanity necessary to defend the charge of adultery as against the ground of indignities.† The distinction is based on the specific intent required for indignities but not for adultery. Adultery is viewed as a more serious moral offense to the marriage, and its defense requires that the person lack sufficient mentality to know what he was doing at the time of the act, or if he did know what he was doing, that he did not know it was wrong. This definition of mental state involves the divorce proceedings in the M'Naghten standard of criminal insanity.[2]

As a grounds for divorce the insanity must be "hopeless and incurable" as determined by medical experts.[1] However, a legal standard, such as mental capacity in ante-nuptial insanity or mental responsibility in the defense to divorce on certain grounds, is not specifically considered.

Thus, there are several degrees of interpretation or definitions of the word "insanity" when used in divorce and annulment proceedings. These become confusing and unclear; judgments often are made on the basis of moral and ethical considerations rather than on medical-legal ones.

Ante-Nuptial Insanity

In annulment proceedings ante-nuptial insanity refers to that state of mind incapable of forming a proper intent or one that could not understand the nature of the proceedings.[1] This definition of insanity is similar to the one utilized in the determination of testamentary capacity or present insanity in criminal proceedings.

Psychiatrists generally have little trouble with the determination of mental capacity. Part of every psychiatric evaluation includes an examination of the mental status wherein the degree of mental capacity of the individual as well as his ability to comprehend the nature of his intended acts is determined. This evaluation is far different from an opinion regarding an individual's degree of responsibility for a certain act as required in criminal law by the M'Naghten formulation.

Thus it is proposed that the name "insanity" used in annul-

---

† See *Manley v. Manley* 192, Pa. Super. 252, 265 (1960).

ment proceedings be changed to mental "incompetency." The state of mind necessary to void a marriage is "mental incompetency," i.e. lack of mental capacity to intend to marry or to comprehend the nature and consequences of the marriage ceremony. "Insanity" should be reserved for the criminal standard of mental irresponsibility.

Postnuptial Insanity as a Defense to Divorce

Insanity is introduced as a defense primarily in cases where divorce is sought on the grounds of cruelty, desertion, or adultery; i.e. serious offenses whereby the defendant is at "fault." The defense claim is lack of mental responsibility at the time of the act, thereby eliminating the "fault." The test of mental responsibility most commonly utilized in these cases is the M'Naghten test as used in criminal proceedings.[2] Thus the psychiatric expert is required to approach the problem by a determination of mental responsibility rather than by a determination of mental capacity as in annulment proceedings.

The question has frequently been asked, "Ought the M'Naghten rules concerning the test of legal insanity in the criminal law also be applied to the law of divorce?" Courts have had great difficulty and have expressed much controversy in resolving this problem, especially with regard to the grounds of cruelty and adultery.

In an early Pennsylvania case[3] it was decided that a woman committing adultery had no good defense of insanity even though the insanity existed at the time of her committing the adultery. This decision erroneously was held to have been the law in Pennsylvania until 1960 when it was overruled by the decision in the *Manley* case.[4] Though the declaration was made by Judge Gibson at that time that insanity did not defend against adultery in a woman, though it might in a man, because of the ethical, moral, social difficulties involved in the "imposing of supposititious offspring." Mrs. Matchin was never declared officially insane. It was generally agreed by all who knew her that she must be insane because she told her husband's kinswoman about her affair with her paramour. Perhaps it was considered insane at that time to do such a thing, but certainly this is not a well accepted criterion for insanity at the present time. It is not really known that Mrs. Matchin was insane at the time of her act, but certainly the definition of insanity used in that case is most erroneous and fallacious. It seems amazing that this decision was maintained for over one hundred years.

A further example of moral judgments in divorce law made in the name of differing degrees of insanity was provided in the very case which overruled the Matchin case.[4] Mr. Manley petitioned for divorce from his wife on the grounds of indignities and later amended the grounds to adultery. Mrs. Manley pleaded insanity. The judgment was that insanity served as a defense against indignities but not against adultery. In essence, because the defendant knew right from wrong, there was no defense on the ground of adultery, but because she lacked intent due to her mental illness, she had a good defense to indignities, for, "such conduct lacks the spirit of hate, estrangement, and malevolence which is the heart of the charge of indignities."[4]

It seems a ridiculous moral rationalization to differentiate between adultery and indignities on the basis of degree of insanity because one offense is "less moral" than the other. Such judgments in the law continue to indicate that adultery is so bad for society that it is essential that one must be totally insane to get away with it and continue in the marriage. (How similar to Judge Gibson's view in *Matchin*.) With regard to insanity as a defense to divorce the following proposals are made:

a. That "insanity" be a defense to any ground for divorce.
b. That insanity be defined in terms of lack of mental ability to intend the offense rather than in terms of the M'Naghten formulation or other test of mental responsibility.
c. That the name "insanity" be reserved in the law for lack of mental responsibility in criminal proceedings; and that the term "unsoundness of mind" be utilized for defense to divorce on any ground. The criterion for establishing "unsoundness of mind" in divorce proceedings is that state of mind that lacks the ability to intend to commit the act charged in the grounds for divorce.

Postnuptial Insanity as Grounds of Divorce

Should postnuptial insanity be included as grounds for divorce? This question has stirred great controversy in the law and has aroused much feeling on both sides of the problem. The ambivalence of social attitudes and mores on this question is reflected in the type of legislation enacted and the nature of judicial decisions handed down.

The traditional argument opposing such legislation was enunciated in a case in Indiana in 1882.

> Insanity is no reason for dissolving the marriage. The statute does not make it one of the grounds for divorce and surely no principle of justice or morality will justify the severance of the marital ties for any such cause. The judgment and conscience revolt at the thought that such a terrible affliction should be deemed cause for separating the wife from the husband. Divorces are granted not because of misfortune, but because of fault. It would be a barbarous code that would allow the wife to put aside the husband because he was stricken by such an awful calamity as the loss of reason.[5]

The uncertainty of this position was reflected by the Pennsylvania legislature in providing for insanity to be a ground for divorce, then completely reversing this provision shortly thereafter. In 1905 a law was passed which declared, "in cases where the husband or wife is a hopeless lunatic or *non compos mentis* the Courts of Common Pleas of the Commonwealth are invested with authority to receive a petition or libel for divorce."[6] In the first case tried under this law, *Bray v. Bray*, the court interpreted the statute as "extending the cause for divorce to a case where either husband or wife is a "hopeless lunatic or *non compos mentis*," thereby judicially affirming hopeless insanity as a new ground for divorce in Pennsylvania.[7] The *Bray* rule persisted until 1907 when two other cases were decided in a contrary opinion.*

---

* *Baughman v. Baughman* 34, Pa. Super. 271 (1907). The court interpreted the statute as merely regulating the procedure in suits for divorce on behalf of an insane libellant and not as creating a new ground for divorce: "To make this misfortune—the greatest that can befall us—the ground of the next greatest wrong and injustice would be truly adding insult and injury to providential misfortune." See also *Johnston v. Johnston* 34, Pa. Super. 606 (1907).

In 1909 the legislature abandoned the notion that the act of 1905 created a new ground for divorce. The legislature apparently bowed to what amounts to a judicial declaration of public policy. In Pennsylvania today there is a provision for divorce on the grounds of incurable insanity, or if the patient has been hospitalized for three years with an unfavorable prognosis by expert psychiatric opinion.

The provision for insanity as a ground for divorce has been made in a gradually increasing number of states. Postnuptial insanity of either husband or wife has been made by statute a grounds of absolute divorce in England and in thirty states in the United States.[1]

In all the jurisdictions wherein insanity is a ground for divorce it must be "incurable insanity." This is a fact to be proved by whatever evidence the law recognizes as competent. It is a matter of expert opinion. It is usually provided that no divorce should be granted for postnuptial insanity unless it is proved beyond a reasonable doubt that it is hopeless, or that the patient has spent or will spend a specific number of years in a mental hospital.

The difficulty with establishing hopeless or incurable insanity as grounds for divorce lies in the definition of the words "insanity" and "hopeless." Who is to say what is "hopeless" in the face of continued research and progress in medical science? With regard to mental illness psychiatrists do not speak of cure, but rather of remissions and exacerbations and consider chronic psychosis a lifelong process.

Thus it is proposed that the word "insanity" be excluded altogether from use as grounds for divorce. The important issue involved in determining whether or not a spouse may be divorced on grounds of insanity is a medical determination of mental illness and not a legal definition of insanity.

It is proposed that the standard be labeled "intractable, unremitting mental illness" as determined by two competent psychiatrists. Furthermore, three years in a state or private mental institution, not necessarily concurrent or without interruption, would be sufficient evidence for the existence of such intractable, unremitting mental illness.

This three-year duration shortens the time in most jurisdictions which is currently from five to ten years. This is appropriate because of the effectiveness of the newer medications in establishing remissions in the more chronic forms of psychosis and mental illness.

Mental illness is chosen because it is a more general term than psychosis; certainly there are many forms of emotional and mental illness other than psychosis which could lead to complete disruption of cohabitational relationship.

Summary and Proposals

The following propositions are presented in an attempt to clarify the confusion and controversy that has existed when insanity has been involved in annulment and divorce proceedings. First, it is proposed that ante-nuptial insanity should not be labeled "insanity" as it is in criminal law, but should be called "mental incompetency," since the requisite state of mind lacks capacity to have been a partner or party to the marriage contract. Secondly, it is recommended that divorce should not be granted if the offender is suffering from mental illness such that he is unable willfully to intend to commit the acts of which he is charged. The mental state vitiating intent as a defense to divorce should be labeled "unsoundness of mind" rather than "insanity."

Thirdly, it is proposed that the term, "intractable, unremitting mental illness," be utilized rather than insanity as a ground for "termination of marriage" (rather than "divorce") when it meets the statutory requirements. Three years in a mental institution or three years following the onset of severe mental illness as determined by two competent psychiatrists should be the standard for termination of marriage on the basis of intractable, unremitting mental illness.

The distinction between "unsoundness of mind" and "intractable, unremitting mental illness" will allow for the stability of marriage which is in keeping with traditional legal attitudes. If one is of unsound mind, one may be incapacitated temporarily and commit acts which would otherwise be grounds for divorce; the party afflicted must be "intractably mentally ill," and not merely "of unsound mind." This concept is in keeping with modern medical opinion of mental illness and encourages treatment and improvement rather than divorce.

These proposed labels in place of "insanity" in annulment and divorce proceedings are not merely different labels for "insanity," but represent different states of mind as determined by psychiatric evaluation consistent with legal criteria. They are presented in an attempt to clarify the confused definition of insanity that pervades Domestic Relations Law, and to bring legal concepts of mental illness up to date with recent advances in psychiatric evaluation and treatment of the mentally ill.

REFERENCES

1. Lindman, F. T. and McIntyre, D. M.: *The Mentally Disabled and the Law*, Chicago, U of Chicago Pr, 1961.
2. M'Naghten's Case, Clark & Fin. 200, 8, Eng. Rep. 718 (1843).
3. *Matchin v. Matchin* 6, Pa. 332, 47, Am. Dec 466 (1847).
4. *Manley v. Manley* 192 Pa. 252, 265 (1960).
5. *Baker v. Baker* 8, Ind 146 (1882).
6. Decker, R. L.: Divorce and insanity in Pennsylvania. *U Pitt L Rev, 20:* 641, 1959.
7. *Bray v. Bray* 15, Dist. 698, 19, Northrum. 167 (1905).

Chapter 17

COMMITMENT PROCEDURES

THE COMMITMENT of persons to hospitals recently has become a complex situation, requiring a number of regulations and safeguards. Traditionally a mentally ill individual could be committed to a hospital on the signature of two physicians with or without court order. In most jurisdictions a patient would need to be found either dangerous to himself or others or in need of hospitalization in order to be committed to a hospital.

Recently, however, involuntary commitments have been challenged by liberal groups seeking to protect the rights of patients. Consequently, interpretations of statutes have precluded involuntary commitment without court sanction except in dire emergencies. No longer will the family be able to "dump" a senile elder member into the state hospital system without a hearing and the possibility of cross-examination of medical testimony.

In Pennsylvania, no hospital will accept a person who is unwilling to be committed unless the court orders the commitment. In the case of an emergency, a ten-day commitment is allowed through the office of the Community Mental Health administrator, who demands evidence of dangerousness of the individual.

Once a person is committed to a state hospital, newer laws have required that he have regular examinations, evaluations and reports prepared for the committing court authority. Also, the patient is required to be instructed of his legal status and be allowed to have an attorney to process his appeal for release if he desires.

Voluntary commitments and admissions continue to be utilized by individuals recognizing that they are sick and in need of treatment. Even voluntary committed patients are required to be notified of their status on a regular basis and may voluntarily leave the hospital after written notice of their intent.

Recently a series of cases has led to a concept of "the right to treatment" of an involuntarily committed patient. That is, a person who is committed to a hospital against his will has the right to adequate treatment within that hospital rather than merely being held there on a custodial basis. Milieu therapy has been found to be insufficient in many cases to meet the requirements of adequate treatment. Chemical therapy; i.e. medication, in addition to milieu therapy may not suffice; rather, active programs for group and individual psychotherapy and rehabilitative measures are required.

The original work on the right to adequate treatment for committed patients was presented in 1960 by Morton Birnbaum, a physician-lawyer who has continued to be active in pursuing implementation of this right. The first significant case was that of *Rouse v. Cameron*[1] in Washington, D.C. Subsequent cases have held that patients committed involuntarily to mental hospitals through noncriminal procedures have a constitutional right to adequate treatment. Recently this decision was upheld in the Federal District Court of Alabama, in which the court ordered, "a treatment program so as to give each of the treatable patients committed to Bryce's facility a realistic opportunity to be cured or to improve his or her mental condition."[2]

According to the judge the constitution requires adequate and effective treatment because without it the hospital is transformed into "a penitentiary where one could be held indefinitely for no convicted offense." The judge said, "The purpose of involuntary hospitalization for treatment purposes is treatment and not mere custodial care or punishment. This is the only justification, from a constitutional standpoint, that allows civil commitments to mental institutions."

The psychiatrist may be called upon to evaluate a person who has been committed to a hospital to determine whether or not he is required to remain in custody. Aside from the recently emerging right to adequate treatment, without which a patient may be discharged from the hospital, the patient also has a right to a writ of habeas corpus, whereby the hospital must show cause why he is required to remain hospitalized. In this instance the patient's lawyer may call in an expert witness, a psychiatrist, to evaluate and examine the patient to determine whether or not such hospitalization is truly required and necessary.

As director of the Forensic Psychiatric Clinic at Temple University several years ago, the author was called upon in about a dozen cases to travel to various hospitals to examine people who had been confined for many years, in some instances. They had raised the issue with the Legal Aid Society or Community Legal Services to determine whether or not they ought to remain in the hospital.

The hospital psychiatrists were delighted to have help; indeed they had been looking for ways of discharging these patients for a long time but were throttled by legal restrictions. They were pleased that the patient had raised the writ of habeas corpus; in fact in some cases had encouraged them to do so. As soon as a lawyer took an interest in the case, the door opened for breaking down the legal barriers to the patient's discharge.

Often the patient was held on a detainer which had little practical significance after years in the hospital, or the psychiatrist in the hospital did not get a response from the judge who had committed the patient and was unable to discharge him without judicial approval. In the majority of cases this was the situation; together, we were able to effect a transfer from the hospital to the community.

In two cases, however, the patient asking for discharge continued to be psychotic and paranoid, and felt that everyone was against him and harming him. In these instances the patient's attorneys were told of the situation to let them know that the patients were still in need of hospitalization and the attorneys should not act on the writs of habeas corpus. Often this is all that is required. The following case is an example of this situation.

> A sixty-eight-year-old single, white woman had written to the Legal Aid Society requesting release from her commitment, since she was not obtaining satisfaction by her own efforts. She had been suffering from a chronic paranoid schizophrenic reaction for many years and had been in the hospital for two years at the time she was evaluated. She claimed that she was

not receiving satisfaction from her doctor and that he was not sympathetic with her need to be released from the hospital. The value of sending a neutral psychiatrist or one representing her counsel to evaluate her had some therapeutic benefit, in that she felt she was understood and that the decision of the psychiatrist was "unbiased."

She was evaluated and the examiner shared with the patient his opinion for her need for continued hospitalization. The information was forwarded to the referring attorney, who then felt more comfortable in not presenting a writ of habeas corpus to release her from commitment.

In only one instance did a "battle" take place. The author testified that the patient ought to be discharged from the hospital and the hospital physicians felt otherwise. Their claim was that they had observed him over a period of time and that my observations were a result of being "conned" by the patient during the examination to believe that he was well enough to be out of the hospital. They cited the long-range approach and the difficulties that he had in living with other people. Nevertheless, the author felt that despite the difficulties, he did not require hospitalization, that he was not dangerous to himself or to others, and that he could well accept and utilize effectively outpatient treatment. During the court appearance, a compromise ensued in which the patient remained in the hospital for a short period of time, then to be followed as an outpatient by the psychiatrist with whom he had worked effectively as an inpatient.

Two prolonged case histories will illustrate some of the problems that a forensic psychiatrist might encounter when handling a commitment matter.

Case Number One

The first is the case of James R., a fifty-two-year-old wealthy corporation executive who had had a twenty-year problem of alcohol abuse. He had spent many months in various hospitals after becoming toxic on alcohol and having fits of violence both toward others and to himself. He had been hospitalized at a private psychiatric hospital and after two weeks was transferred to the regional state hospital where he had spent three months under a ninety-day commitment. He had petitioned to leave the hospital after ninety days, claiming he had been cured and he was planning to return to work and would be able to function without the use of alcohol. His wife signed a counter petition to keep him in the hospital until he was definitely cured such that she could count on his returning effectively to the household and to a productive life.

The hospital authorities felt that Mr. R. ought to remain in the hospital for a prolonged period of time, that his prognosis was hopeless, and that he would never be much improved even after years of hospitalization. This being the case, the author felt he ought to be given the chance to work on the outside, with an AA program with frequent outpatient treatment, which he was able to afford, and to take the chance that he would be able to stay off alcohol. In this instance it was important to show the court how his life situations had changed and that he would not be likely to return to the use of alcohol.

We know, however, that there is a likely recurrence because of the habituation and addiction one has toward alcohol after such a chronic history. My main plea was that if the prognosis were so hopeless, there appeared little sense in keeping him in the hospital if he could not benefit from his hospital stay. In this case Mr. R. was allowed to be discharged from the hospital, obtain private treatment from another psychiatrist and return to work.

Case Number Two

John F., a forty-three-year-old French electronics engineer who had been hospitalized for an acute psychotic reaction, was seeking discharge from the hospital at the expiration of his sixty-day commitment. His wife felt that he was still psychotic and ought to remain in the hospital for a prolonged period of time. The physicians at the hospital also agreed that his condition warranted prolonged inpatient treatment. Mr. F. had had a previous hospitalization the year before, under similar circumstances of an acute psychotic breakdown, and had left the hospital prematurely, did not cooperate in outpatient treatment, nor on medication and had a relapse shortly before his second hospitalization.

The author had been called in by his attorney to testify in his behalf at the hearing. After examining Mr. F., it was found that he was indeed chronically ill and in need of prolonged hospitalization. This was related at the hearing with a suggestion that he be reevaluated in sixty days and at that time a more definitive disposition could be made. His disappointment in the delay, coupled with his paranoid delusional system, prompted him to elope from the hospital three days after the hearing. He fled to France and has not returned to this country.

One of the difficulties involved in the latter case was the support he received from a lay group headed by a woman who felt that commitment proceedings in America were cruel and that John was not mentally ill and should not be made to stay in a hospital against his will. She accepted his delusional system as reality and supported his outrageous demands that he made upon his wife and family as being "perhaps extreme but not crazy."

It should be pointed out very clearly that commitment to a hospital does not in every state mean loss of competency; i.e. a person who is committed has the same rights and privileges he had prior to his commitment to the hospital. In some states, however, there is an automatic loss of rights with the commitment to the hospital. These rights usually are reinstated when the person is discharged from the hospital. In some cases a hearing must be held in order to reinstate competency to manage one's own affairs even after discharge from a hospital.

Most of the questions that psychiatrists ask in conferences are concerned with commitment procedures, especially the mechanism by which a patient may be hospitalized against his will when he is examined in the emergency room of a general hospital. It is difficult to discuss these mechanisms in a single book covering general considerations, since the mechanisms differ from state to state. Many of the questions are asked by residents about medical patients or surgical patients who become acutely psychotic and are in need of transfer to a psychiatric facility. Others refer to patients seen in the emergency room of the hospital on a weekend or an evening when the patient has posed a threat or a danger to his family, or to himself, or to others. The question is always, "What do we do?" "Where do we hospitalize him?" or, "Can we be sued for hospitalizing him against his will?"

The answers to these questions primarily depend upon the regulations and statutes in the various jurisdictions. As a general rule, a physician acting in good faith to protect the interest of his patient, the health and welfare of others, may feel the need to hospitalize in order to segregate an individual for his protection and his treatment. Acting in good faith, it is unlikely that a physician or a psychiatrist will be successfully sued for "false imprisonment" or for negligence in the care of his patient.

Occasionally the questions are more sophisticated and require intimate knowledge of the various operational procedures within a city or county. Often the laws themselves tie the hands of the psychiatrist attempting to practice good medicine and effectively treat his patient. In many cases the law will disallow the patient from being hospitalized and necessitate either his going free or indirectly being incarcerated through criminal means. A court may be required to send him to the hospital for proper medical care.

The effect of these newer laws and regulations is to safeguard the patient's and the citizen's individual legal rights while jeopardizing his medical rights. However, one judge stated that a person has no medical rights without legal rights, and most physicians are quite aware of the classic instances in which a person incarcerated in the local prison in order to uphold his legal rights successfully killed himself. Such a tragedy may have been averted had the patient been sent directly to the hospital instead. In such an instance the patient died with all of his legal rights intact and preserved. Thus, involuntary commitment has become a comprehensive, complex problem, requiring caution and care and appropriate medical-legal consultation.

REFERENCES

1. *Rouse v. Cameron*, 125, US App. DC 366, 373 F.2d 451 (1967).
2. *Wyatt v. Stickney*, 325 F. Supp. 781; 334 F. Supp. 1341; 344 S. Supp. 373; 344 F. Supp. 387 (M.D. Ala. 1971-1972).

Chapter 18

THE PSYCHIATRIST AND THE EVALUATION OF TRAUMA

THE PSYCHIATRIST'S ROLE in the evaluation of traumatic injury has been gradually increasing. Traditionally the psychiatrist had been called when there was a question of a traumatic neurosis following physical trauma leading to physical injury with concomitant emotional difficulties. This role has been expanded to include evaluation of individuals who have emotional illness following trauma where there is no touching and no concomitant physical illness. The role has been extended to workmen's compensation cases where traditionally a touching had occurred during an injury at work. Currently, however, a purely emotional or psychiatric condition may arise from the work situation with no physical injury.

Workmen's compensation evaluation is a branch of the general field of psychiatric examination for traumatic injury. Often the person to be evaluated has sustained, or claims to have sustained, an injury while at work with resulting emotional problems. The opportunity for deception is great in this situation since there is a built-in mechanism for rewarding illness and damage, whereas in general tort actions one has to prove negligence and responsibility as well as damage. In the workmen's compensation area a person receives his percentage of disability and has a continuous review by psychiatrist. Often the original physical damage has been healed, leaving a residual of emotional problems which need evaluation and treatment.

It is the function of the psychiatrist to determine medically whether or not this damage is related to and caused by the origi-

---

This chapter is modified in part from material originally published in the volume on *Psychic Injuries* contained in the series *Courtroom Medicine*, © 1975. Matthew Bender & Company, N.Y.

nal injury or whether it is due to completely isolated and unrelated events occurring in the patient's life. One of the problems that may arise is the tendency to almost automatically relate what the psychiatrist observes and what he learns from the history. Thus it is especially important to take a careful and complete history to determine whether or not there are other sources for emotional pain, or aggravation of original illness, that are not due to, or related to, the original trauma. Because one suffers does not necessarily mean that the suffering is due to the one injury that he wishes to talk about.

Most psychiatrists are not attuned to the preparation of material fitting into percentage of disability. It is very difficult, for example, to decide how disabled is a person who has a schizophrenic reaction. Can he work at some type of job? Can he work at the particular job that he had at the time of his original injury? Is he 70 percent, 85 percent or 50 percent disabled? Mostly we do not think in terms of percentages and this may cause attorneys great consternation in attempting to pin the psychiatrist down to specific percentages.

The AMA has prepared a guide to the evaluation of permanent impairment in mental illness, published in 1971.[1] They classify clinical types of mental disorders in the following terms:

1. mental deficiency, mental retardation
2. personality disorders
3. sociopathic personality disturbance, psychopathic personality
4. psychoneuroses or neuroses
5. psychoses
6. chronic brain syndrome

Disability is presented in terms of impairment of the whole man and percentages 0 to 15 percent, 20 to 45 percent, 50 to 85 percent, and 95 percent are given. In personality disorders, the guide states, "Permanent impairment would rarely exceed 5 percent on a longitudinal basis." For sociopathic personality the guide suggests that it is unlikely that the psychiatric impairment would ever exceed 45 percent. The guide for psychoneurotic conditions is much more complex and the psychoses also are spelled out fairly clearly as to the extent of disability to the whole man. The severity of chronic brain syndromes suggests the degree of disability.

The forensic psychiatrist may be asked to evaluate the validity of an illness, whether malingering is involved, and to aid in the follow-up evaluation of persons claiming mental and emotional difficulties due to previous trauma. That prior trauma may be negligent care of a patient by another doctor resulting in damage and prompting a malpractice suit. Often patients who claim damage due to medical negligence have related emotional components that require professional evaluation and treatment.

For further understanding of the medical aspects of psychic injuries, a few concepts and terms require brief discussion.

Hysteria, as used generally means a panic state with shouting, screaming, crying and uncontrollable behavior. "She becomes hysterical." The *hysterical personality* disorder usually refers to a woman who is attractive, seductive, charming and histrionic in her relationships with others. She tends to exaggerate difficulties and show emotional lability, excitability and self-dramatization. These individuals are immature, self-centered, vain and usually dependent on others.

A third use of the word hysteria relates to the *hysterical neurosis,* which is characterized by an "involuntary psychogenic loss or disorder of function." This is a mental illness of neurotic proportions and consists of two types: the *conversion* type and *dissociative* type. The individual with hysteria has converted his emotional conflicts into physical symptoms which may provide secondary gain by allowing sympathy or relief of anxiety. The classic example is the pilot in wartime who develops a paralyzed arm and cannot fly and does not have to face his fears directly. The *dissociative* type relates to an altered state of consciousness with such symptoms as amnesia, somnambulism (sleepwalking) fugue state and multiple personality. A typical example of this type of dissociative reaction is the individual who leads a double life; i.e. he has left one situation without remembering and has started a second life in a different locale. He may live it for five or ten years or more, or indefinitely without realizing he had a past life. *The Three Faces of Eve* by Corbett Thigpen and Hervey M. Checkley illustrates such a dissociative or multiple personality state.

The conversion symptoms seen in the hysterical personality or hysterical neurosis must be differentiated from *psychophysiological reactions*. Many of the symptoms may appear similar in the structure of the body affected. Careful evaluation and use of hypnosis or drugs may aid in the differentiation between a true psychophysiological reaction to stress or to the hysterical conversion symptoms.

Secondary gain is seen primarily in individuals with psychoneurotic problems who respond to injury in an exaggerated manner. Their lack of function resolves a more important problem for them of which they are not aware (i.e. it resides in the unconscious) but which gives them a feeling of relief of anxiety.

Malingering in psychiatric terms is lying. There is no psychiatric concept of malingering which is not conscious fabrication. A malingerer is one who is responding to an injury by a falsified deceptive set of symptoms. It is conscious exaggeration or fabrication of symptoms as opposed to an unconscious attempt at resolution of conflicts.

Post-Traumatic Neurosis

This is a very specific syndrome or collection of symptoms following trauma. The post-traumatic neurosis is not a usual response to trauma, but only one of many. The classical description of the traumatic neurosis is given by Modlin[2] who lists the following symptoms:

1. anxiety
2. muscular tension
3. irritability
4. impaired concentration and memory
5. repetitive nightmares
6. sexual inhibition
7. social withdrawal

In most of the cases he studied, the syndrome was a short-lived one and usually promptly resolved. A person may have a prolonged response to injury that may be related to the injury and caused by it, but it may not be a post-traumatic neurosis.

It is important to differentiate the various kinds of responses an individual can have to stress and be certain that our label is identifiable by other psychiatrists in a standardized labeling procedure. Otherwise we may have psychiatrists calling the same condition by different labels in order to produce a specific legal result. Robitscher[3] lists a number of labels which all refer to post-traumatic neurosis: neurotic neurosis, neurosis following trauma, triggered neurosis, personal injury neurosis, occupational neurosis, stress reaction, combat fatigue, shell shock, compensation neurosis and secondary gain neurosis. He feels that we can clarify the situation by dealing with the cases in three categories, as follows:

1. *Traumatic neurosis:* a healthy individual became mentally ill as a result of an overwhelming stress;
2. *Compensation or triggered neurosis:* the individual had a latent illness triggered or precipitated by the trauma and held onto by the patient for largely unconscious reasons;
3. *Malingering:* The individual consciously deceives.

The three reactions may be restated as follows: first, the injury may have led to an emotional reaction called neurosis, psychosis or other form of emotional entity or disorder which did not precede the illness. Secondly, the illness may have precipitated or aggravated an underlying emotional difficulty or disorder. Third, the injury had no recognizable or identifiable effect upon the individual except as he complains about it.

We must differentiate between subjective complaints and objective symptoms. In physical medicine this task is much easier, but in psychiatry there are objective findings which can be listed to which patients are not particularly attuned. One of these is the repetition of dreams relating to the trauma itself. Another is muscular tension and a third is irritability noted by others. Vague complaints over a long period of time by individuals are not necessarily neurotic. Also, any complaint that does not have an identifiable cause in physical examination does not necessarily mean that the symptom is caused by emotional factors. It may be completely fabricated. Also, some people are more sensitive to certain stresses and stimuli than others and will complain as they may have complained about other conditions earlier in their lives.

Examination for Psychic Injury

The psychiatrist called by the plaintiff's attorney will be looking for a relationship between the accident, or trauma, and the emotional symptoms. It is suggested that he look for causes other than the trauma so that he can explain symptoms which occur that may not be a part of the traumatic injury syndrome.

The psychiatrist must initially put the plaintiff at ease and must encourage him to be as open and honest as he possibly can. He must elicit the information about the trauma as clearly as he is able and in as great detail as possible. The plaintiff should talk about the trauma or the accident and the symptoms that he experienced following the accident. It is important to note whether or not there was unconsciousness following the trauma; whether or not there was an amnesia or memory loss for events prior to and following the traumatic event. These questions may be interspersed or asked at a later time. The author prefers to have the plaintiff tell his story in his own words and then go back and ask questions to fill in the gaps.

A list of symptoms that the plaintiff currently experiences is very important. How do these differ from symptoms he experienced directly after the accident; what changes has he noted from the time of the trauma to the present? What else has been occurring in the individual's life that might influence or affect his personality or his emotional state? Thus, a careful present history is essential.

Past history is also considered to be a significant part of the examination and interview because one must determine whether or not this reaction was a pattern that the plaintiff had experienced previously. Had there been prior trauma? What was the individual's reaction to previous stress in his life? Can this information help us to establish current patterns which otherwise might not be as well understood?

Also, was there history of previous damage due to prior trauma that continued to the instant accident, was not caused by it, but might have been aggravated by it?

We need a family history, educational history, vocational history, past medical history, specifically obtaining information on previous injuries, periods of unconsciousness, use or abuse of alcohol, tobacco and drugs, previous operations, fractures, periods of hospitalization, or consultation with psychiatrists or psychologists. In essence, we need to develop a pretraumatic personality base for the individual to try and establish what kind of a person on which this trauma was inflicted. Detailed information regarding the plaintiff's interests, behavior patterns, hobbies, plans, goals, eating and sleeping patterns, work and school record must be obtained. Also, we need to consider statements by relatives, friends, neighbors, employers, physicians and relevant others regarding past history and how it differs from present conditions. This is true for psychiatric examinations by both plaintiff and defense psychiatrists.

A *mental status examination* is then conducted. This is very important in evaluating for malingering, determining consistency of story, and determining presence of psychosis, neurosis or personality disorder. We look for demeanor, dress, neatness, consistency, cooperation, presentation of materials, speech impediments, observation of movements, whether feigned, exaggerated or normal; we note inconsistencies in psychomotor features. We notice the method and manner in which the individual relates his story: are there gaps in memory? Is he oriented to time, place and person? Are there features of hallucinations or delusions? Is he out of touch with reality? Is he flexible in his abstraction of proverbs? Can he calculate properly? What is the estimate of his intelligence and what kind of personality does he demonstrate?

A *tentative diagnostic impression* is usually arrived at following the first interview with a consideration of recommendations for further evaluation and/or treatment. Further evaluation may include repeat visits, psychological testing, neurological tests, blood tests, brain wave test and other medical tests. Treatment may include psychotherapy, group therapy, family therapy, medication, hospital care or other treatment.

Consultation with attorney is very important for obtaining the proper records of previous hospitalizations and medical examinations, other psychiatric evaluations or psychological testing. Does this individual need a comprehensive battery of psychological tests, and if so, for what purposes? Does he need a sodium amytal interview to help erase the amnesia and regain his memory? Does he need hypnotic interviews? Does he need any physical tests such as electroencephalogram or a lumbar puncture (spinal tap)? Does he need a neurological examination or other physical examinations or chemical tests of the blood or other body fluids? Are there considerations in his history which might account for the symptoms that he demonstrates or of which he complains? How are these to be considered or weighted with the traumatic event? What are the objective signs noted to corroborate subjective symptoms? What "evidence" can be presented by the psychiatrist to support or negate the claim?

In evaluating a plaintiff for defendant's counsel, it is important for the psychiatrist to be certain he has all the reports and evaluations available to him before his examination. In essence, he is called in to rebut the findings of another psychiatrist (or psychiatrists) and he must know what that psychiatrist has said before he can properly or effectively rebut the specifics of the plaintiff's psychiatrist's evaluations and conclusions.

It should be emphasized that no two people see a patient or plaintiff in the same way. Each psychiatrist has his own frame of reference and has a subjectivity about his evaluation which colors his view of the symptoms and his interpretation of findings. Occasionally two psychiatrists approaching the problem from opposite ends will observe the same features but will come to different interpretations. The plaintiff may present a different picture to each psychiatrist in order to gain his most favorable ends. The other psychiatrist may not be wrong in his interpretation, merely different. He may have a different focus or avoid or overlook certain features which make the diagnosis and the interpretation more obvious. The important feature here is the *communication,* first between the plaintiff and the psychiatrist; second between the psychiatrist and the attorney for whom he is examining the plaintiff, and third, between the psychiatrist and the court if expert testimony is required.

We have already shown the need for and extent of materials for examination and methods for obtaining as much information as is available from the plaintiff. A very important consideration is the communication at the attorney-physician conference during which is shared specific need for further information, strategies of presenting material and focus on the data collected. During this conference the attorney must spell out to the psychiatrist what is expected of him, a definite opinion regarding the plaintiff, his symptoms and their relation to the accident or trauma. The psychiatrist must in turn let the attorney know how definite he can be in what areas of the case and where he anticipates weakness in his testimony. Anticipation of thoughtful cross-examination is quite helpful in preparing both attorney and expert psychiatric witness.

Finally, the communication of the psychiatrist in court as an expert witness should be clear, credible and based on reasonable medical certainty. Any psychiatric testimony can be effectively attacked by careful, thoughtful cross-examination. The psychiatric opinion, while definitive, is based on evidence that is not absolute and the psychiatric witness should expect to be interrogated in areas that weaken his position. He must identify these areas in advance and be prepared to respond in a manner that may weaken his final conclusions, but not destroy his opinion or his credibility as an expert.

Attorney Evaluates Plaintiff

At this point, it will be helpful to discuss an example of a client involved in an accident seeking legal advice. The client enters the lawyer's office and complains of headaches, dizziness, anxiety, following an automobile accident three weeks previously. He said he had been hospitalized for one week following a period of unconsciousness at the scene of the accident and a diagnosis of cerebral concussion was made. He demonstrates memory loss for the actual event of the accident. He describes a blow to the head with a lump, but skull X rays are negative for fracture and no positive neurological findings are noted. In essence he has had a physical injury to the head with minimal brain involvement, called a concussion. He describes symptoms which may be related to the trauma to his brain and he has obvious emotional ramifications.

The astute attorney wishes to know more and looks for evidence of anxiety, tremulousness, nervousness, erratic movements of the hand, gait, instability of physical movements, and asks questions about social, family life and behavior. He also asks medical history of similar symptoms, sleep patterns, eating habits, working patterns. It is likely that this individual has suffered a post-concussion syndrome. In this case he has had actual physical involvement of the brain with classical emotional symptoms, usually labeled post-concussion syndrome, sometimes post-traumatic syndrome following concussion, or even post-traumatic neurosis. It is very clear that a post-traumatic neurosis is a specific series of symptoms which follow trauma but does not necessarily involve physical damage or even brain involvement.

It is important to note that the "magical" label *post-traumatic neurosis* is a relatively rare occurrence following trauma and there are a number of other post-traumatic symptoms or syndromes that occur that may also be compensable and require psychiatric evaluation. There are a number of combinations of traumatic reactions that may occur of which the attorney ought to be aware. The client may have sustained physical damage to his body, not necessarily to his brain, and have an emotional reaction following the trauma. The damage may have been slight or it may have been severe. It may be to his extremities or his torso or his head. His emotional reaction may depend upon the severity of the physical damage and the location of that damage. For example, if a surgeon injures his hand, the emotional reaction will be more significant than if the same injury occurred to a psychiatrist. Emotional reaction will also be dependent upon the pretraumatic personality configuration of the client. Will the emotional reaction take the form of depression, anxiety, hysterical reaction, phobic symptoms, obsessive-compulsive reaction or even a psychotic reaction? Will there merely be an aggravation of an individual's personality disorder because of the physical injury? Everyone will regress a bit with physical injury whether it incapacitates or hospitalizes him, or merely reminds him that he is in pain and is not free of symptoms as he was prior to the accident. The regression may take the form of excessive dependency, inability to work effectively, social withdrawal or even depression.

Certainly with physical damage to the head and even slight impairment of the brain tissue by means of concussion, the emotional reaction will be more serious than if the head or brain was not involved. A concussion usually leaves no lasting residual on the brain tissue but is merely a bruise of the brain causing unconsciousness, memory loss and some residual anxiety. However, since the brain is such a sensitive organ about which one has great feelings of insecurity when it is injured, the emotional reaction is likely to be quite serious. Other physical symptoms may also linger, causing aggravation of emotional reaction. Headaches or dizziness may be present when they were not previously. These symptoms may incapacitate a person and keep him from working or functioning effectively.

How can one determine whether these "subjective" symptoms are emotionally derived or caused by the insult to the brain, or are made up by the patient in order to gain compensation?

One cannot always be sure but there are means of testing these symptoms, especially over time. Usually following a concussion the symptoms will clear rather rapidly so that no brain damage is detected. Electroencephalogram, skull X ray, lumbar puncture, brain scan, should all be within normal limits. Because the physical tests to detect an organic etiology to the symptoms are negative does not necessarily mean that the symptoms are based on emotional instability or psychiatric causation. It may be that the individual is malingering or exaggerating his symptoms because of his own personality problems. Also, the symptoms may be hysterical; i.e. based on a psychoneurotic problem of which the patient is not aware.

These subjective symptoms of headache and dizziness following concussion in an automobile accident are fairly common and may be prolonged by unduly delayed litigation and by promises that settlement or compensation will be greater if the individual is "sicker." It is the responsibility of the attorney to his client to keep him from abusing the system by aggravating his medical symptoms. The attorney must be aware of the type of individual that he is dealing with to know whether certain tactics or strategies will aggravate his symptoms or help alleviate the difficulties he is experiencing.

A person need not be injured physically in an accident to show an emotional response to the accident. The accident itself may or may not be traumatic; that is, it may not result in emotional scars or emotional damage to the victim.

A seventeen-year-old high school senior was a passenger in an automobile that was struck by another car at an intersection. The driver was injured by sustaining a fractured leg, a series of fractured ribs against the steering wheel and had some internal damage requiring abdominal surgery. The passenger in the front seat hit her head on the windshield and suffered a concussion with cuts and bruises. One of the passengers in the back seat was thrown clear of the automobile and died as a result of the injuries sustained. The individual in question was also in the back seat and was not injured physically, and showed no emotional sequelae to the accident. He showed no abnormal phobic symptoms about driving or riding in cars. He was saddened about the death of his friend and mourned appropriately, but did not become overly depressed. He showed no evidence for post-traumatic neurosis or pathological emotional response. Emphasis is placed on the word *pathological* because everyone in such a situation will *normally* show an emotional reaction to that trauma, to that accident.

That is not the significant feature of the injuries sustained. What is important is a pathological or unusual or prolonged emotional response which is not normal. The driver sustaining the abdominal injuries and the broken ribs also showed no serious pathological emotional response to the trauma since it was his contention that the fault lay on the part of the driver who hit his car. He was also saddened by the death of his friend but did not feel responsible nor did he mourn unduly long with depressive symptoms.

The front seat passenger sustaining the concussion and memory loss also showed a post-traumatic depressive reaction with phobic symptoms. This pathological emotional response took the form of phobia for driving and prolonged depression over the death of her friend. Psychiatric treatment was necessary to help her regain her pretraumatic personality configuration and to clear up the psychoneurotic symptoms that were caused by this accident.

Thus in the one accident there are four responses: one is death, one is a physical injury with brain involvement, leading to a classical post-traumatic neurotic condition with phobic and depressive symptoms. The third and fourth reveal no pathological emotional responses, though one was physically injured and the other was not.

On the other hand, there may be a case of an individual who shows no physical injury during the accident but who subsequently emerges with a post-traumatic neurosis of the classical type. Similarly, there may be a post-traumatic emotional reaction not as serious as a psychoneurosis or psychosis which may be a result of an accident in which no physical damage was sustained. Thus, no phobic symptoms or hysterical symptoms were noted but an aggravation of one's passivity and dependency following an accident was noted in which no physical damage was sustained.

When to Call the Psychiatrist

How does an attorney know when his client requires the services of a forensic psychiatrist to evaluate emotional damage or psychic injury? Often attorneys will call a psychiatrist when their medical doctors detect illness without organic components or without being able to determine for certain the cause of symptoms which have no relationship to medical, organic or anatomical counterparts. The psychiatrist then will be called in as a rule-out phenomenon; i.e. all other forms of illness or reasons for the symptoms have been ruled out by the neurologist, the internist or the orthopaedic surgeon and, because the patient still has complaints, he must have an emotional illness. That is a dangerous way of approaching mental illness because it is from the back door and by negative results. In my opinion, psychic injury must show positive evidence for emotional damage rather than negative evidence for physical or anatomical structural damage. It may be that in many cases the individual suffering these symptoms without evidence of medical etiology or causation does have a bona fide emotional illness or psychic injury, but a competent psychiatrist is required to make a positive diagnosis, rather than to assume or presume that there must be emotional illness because one cannot explain the symptoms by any other reason.

Once the psychiatrist is called by plaintiff's attorney he must be told exactly what had occurred, what positive medical findings there are, why the psychiatrist is being called, and what the attorney expects or hopes he will find. Other factors in a person's life may be very important to the development of symptoms which might originally be presumed to have occurred as a result of the injury rather than occurring independently, though following the accident. A case in point will illustrate the importance of taking a thorough and careful social history as well as occasionally interviewing the patient in the presence of his or her attorney.

This case is that of a teenage girl who was hit over the head in a fight, resulting in a change of her personality; she did poorly in school, was more irritable at home and had periods of moodiness and depression. Her attorney was hoping to correlate her change in mood with the traumatic blow to the head which resulted in a bona fide concussion with neurological sequelae shortly after the accident, but which remitted completely soon thereafter.

Psychiatric examination of the youngster, both alone and in the company of her mother, revealed that she had a difficult relationship with her father, who was an alcoholic and mistreated her mother. In addition she was having difficulty with a boyfriend and also with her other siblings. There was one suicidal attempt shortly after the accident which was thought to be related to the accident and to her changing mood.

Careful interviewing, however, revealed that this attempt was due to her depressive reaction following her mother's heart attack which had occurred in the intervening time. She was depressed primarily because her mother had become an invalid and she was required to assume all the responsibilities at home. Having her attorney present at that interview was indeed helpful in conveying the significance of the family dynamics and the family's problems relating to her change in mood. He became convinced that it would be impossible for the psychiatrist to state that the accident had caused her change of mood or even affected it in light of the overwhelming difficulties which emerged during the interview but which he had not previously been able to ascertain.

Positive evidence for emotional illness therefore is one criterion which needs to be established. The second criterion that needs to be developed is the evidence that this emotional difficulty is in fact related to and caused by the injury or accident in question. As revealed in the foregoing case, there was indeed mood change, depression and emotional illness, but it was not possible to determine the exact etiology of this mood change. In fact, it is more likely that the depression was due to her change in life-style for reasons independent of the accident though they followed the time of the accident.

Examining the Plaintiff for Defense Counsel

This examination poses several other issues which need to be discussed. First, cooperation between the defense counsel and plaintiff's counsel should be achieved so that the examination is conducted at a mutually suitable time. The plaintiff's counsel may be present during the examination or may not be, depending upon his choice. Some psychiatrists prefer to examine a patient by themselves and will not examine an individual with someone else in the room. The author has found that the presence of another individual who is noninterfering is not a distraction and it does not significantly affect the psychiatric interview. Often plaintiff's attorney or his representative can be helpful in providing more information than otherwise available.

However, it is helpful to require all of the reports that have been prepared and made available to defense counsel before seeing the plaintiff. The reason for this is to aid in asking specific questions and confronting him with questions that may provide inconsistencies or inaccuracies that will be needed in evaluating his claim of injury.

Start an examination for defense counsel with the plaintiff by telling him who you are, whom you represent, what will be done with the words that he utters in the interview, and what you will do with the examination and report. He has a right to know this and it is a matter of his informed consent to talk with you.

It should be stated at the outset that psychiatrists are trained to find or evaluate mental illness. It is much more difficult for a psychiatrist to determine the absence of mental illness than the presence of it. Thus, examining for the defense counsel is much more difficult and poses a greater challenge to the forensic psychiatrist. There may be hostility or defensiveness on the part of the plaintiff who is afraid he is going to be trapped or excessively tested by the psychiatrist for the defense. It is up to the psychiatrist to put the plaintiff at ease and to assure him that he is not out to trap him or to trick him, but merely to do his best job in evaluating the claims the plaintiff is making about his state of mind and his mental condition.

Often the plaintiff will be deceptive, sometimes will lie or malinger during the examination. It is normal to assume the plaintiff will put his best legal foot forward; that is, to present his symptoms in as clear a manner as he can in order to convince the examining psychiatrist that he is entitled to damages. It is important for the psychiatrist examining the plaintiff for the defense to be able to look for, if not find, alternative solutions or reasons for the condition of the plaintiff. One of these conditions may be malingering or deception.

How does a psychiatrist determine whether a person is malingering about certain symptoms? One method is to do what other physicians do and that is, rule out. If the plaintiff comes in with a story of symptoms that do not fit emotional conditions observed during the examination, then there is a discrepancy between the signs and symptoms of the alleged illness. If, for example, a person says he is unable to work following an accident at work, one has to determine the reason why he is unable to work. If it is a bona fide medical or mental or emotional condition, then there ought to be positive evidence for such a condition. If no such evidence is found, the suspicion of malingering or deception is raised.

The Psychiatric Consultant

The psychiatric consultant in any of these cases must have an atmosphere of credibility about him as his most important tool. Attorneys who wish to purchase the services of psychiatrists because they are good plaintiff's witnesses or defense witnesses are foolish. They run the risk of buying psychiatric testimony without the value of its credibility. Lawyers soon get to know whom to call for plaintiff's cases and whom for defense cases. There are psychiatrists who will invariably find something wrong with anyone who has been involved in an accident, and others who will be more careful to assign a mental illness only if one is present and only if there is positive evidence for its existence. Some for the defense will be hardened to the claims of many individuals and will, based on their experiences, personality and other biases, be likely not to find evidence for mental illness, sometimes because they don't wish to find it.

It is extremely important for an effective forensic psychiatrist to be able to testify on both sides of the fence (but not, of course, in the same case). He should be comfortable in testifying for defense counsel as well as for plaintiff's counsel. This gives him the opportunity of anticipating the kinds of questions or cross-examination that will occur for whichever side he testifies.

Lawyers, of course, are wise to find someone who has a good track record in previous testimony so that they can have the best chance of success for their side. Others would rather have the benefit of an honest open psychiatric opinion that would give them some reliable indication about the value of their case and how to proceed.

REFERENCES

1. Guides to the evaluation of permanent impairment: Mental illness. Chicago, AMA, 1971.
2. Modlin, H. C.: The post-accident anxiety syndrome: Psychosocial aspects. *Am J Psychiat, 123*:8, 1967.
3. Robitscher, J. B.: *Pursuit of Agreement: Psychiatry and the Law.* Philadelphia, Lippincott, 1966.

SECTION IV

THE LAW AND THE PSYCHIATRIST

THIS FINAL SECTION consists of only two chapters dealing with ethical and legal issues confronting the psychiatrist. All psychiatrists and attorneys should be aware of the practical application of such concepts as confidentiality, privilege, informed consent and the duty the psychiatrist owes his patient. The section is geared more perhaps for the practicing psychiatrist than for the attorney, but does give the practicing attorney a chance to understand some of the problems faced by psychiatrists in their practice of medicine. Hopefully the greater insights obtained will lead to improvement in our mutual efforts to aid clients and patients, and to promote and encourage progress in this increasingly complex interdisciplinary field.

Chapter 19

LEGAL RESPONSIBILITIES OF THE PSYCHIATRIST

Malpractice and the Psychiatrist

THERE ARE TWO AREAS in malpractice where the psychiatrist may be involved. One is as an expert witness in a suit involving another physician or psychiatrist, and the other is as a defendant in a suit against himself. The primary basis of liability in malpractice acts is the deviation from the standard of conduct of a responsible and prudent physician. The basis for action in malpractice is negligence. In order for a malpractice claim to be effective, the plaintiff, i.e. the one who is complaining about the damage done to him, must be able to prove the existence of four factors, (1) *duty* due the patient by the physician; there is an established relationship between the physician and the plaintiff-patient, in which the physician owes the patient a duty. This duty may exist if the physician treats the patient by advice or medication, but it does not exist after merely an examination or evaluation and a referral to another doctor. The duty is not related to compensation or collection of fee. (2) *Dereliction* of this duty by the physician toward the patient, a deviation in the care of the patient. (3) *Direct* causation by the dereliction of duty or (4) *damage* to the patient-plaintiff.

Thus for a malpractice claim to be effective there must be *damage* to the patient which was caused *directly* by the *dereliction* of the *duty* the physician owed the patient. There can be no active negligence without all four d's involved. Generally a physician is liable for bad practice resulting in injury to the patient. He must exercise a degree of skill and judgment comparable to that possessed by others in his profession or specialty. The physician is not liable for injury, however, if he exercises the required degree of skill and care. Where there are several accepted methods of treatment, the doctor may adopt any one of them, even though it is not the one most widely used. In these cases of alleged malpractice, an expert witness is required to present the standards of care in the community. However, in some cases the abuse is so evident even to a layman, that no expert is required. These are cases of *res ipsa loquitur,* a Latin phrase meaning "the thing speaks for itself." This phrase is significant in malpractice cases in which expert medical testimony is not required but that the injury is obvious even to a layman. In effect, this theory shifts to the doctor and the burden of proof in defending himself, where otherwise the burden is on the patient to prove that the doctor is at fault.

Informed Consent

The concept of informed consent is also an important one for the psychiatrist to understand. That is, he must explain to his patient, preferably in writing, that the patient understands the nature and consequences of any procedure which is to be performed upon him. This is usually more significant in general medicine, where surgery and other operations may result in limitations of function or other aftereffects. In psychiatry, however, the use of medication or electroshock therapy or even hospitalization must be explained to the patient so that he understands the risks he is taking by accepting the mode of treatment offered by the physician.

No guarantee of results can be made or should be made by the psychiatrist; the psychiatrist is not expected to anticipate or foresee the unexpected. One also is not expected to convey fear to the patient by explaining in every detail the rare side effects that could occur from the medication or procedure. This method would probably frighten the patient to the point where he would not accept the medication and the possibility of improvement by an accepted and appropriate medication for his illness. See Chapter 20 for further discussion of informed consent.

Pain and Suffering

In many recent cases "pain and suffering" or "mental trauma" is often added to other physical damage and is included in the basic amount of damages. The *Wall Street Journal* recently ran an article in which a New York housewife was burned by X rays while being treated for bursitis. Later a doctor warned her the burn scars could turn into cancer. The woman sued the radiologist who burned her and collected 25,000 dollars in damages. Ten thousand dollars was for the burns, the other 15,000 dollars compensated her for her "cancerophobia," the neurotic fear of cancer, she said she developed because of the burns. In summarizing the problem of the cancerophobic patient, the Appeals Court maintained, "Freedom from mental disturbance is now a protected interest of the state."

In a study conducted by Bellamy[1] involving liability of psychiatrists in malpractice suits (1946-1961), in the Appellate Court (only 1 out of 100 cases reaches the Appellate Court), he found there were eighteen psychiatric claims with thirteen psychiatrists involved. The types of risks encountered included:

1. problems of treatment—nine (7 involved electroshock therapy)
2. problems of commitment—six
3. problems of suicide—one
4. miscellaneous—two

Further, he cited the following areas of difficulty for the psychiatrist:

1. implied promise of cure invites a claim for alleged breach of warranty;
2. suit for assault and battery may be brought for alleged unenlightened consent.

The contention of the law is that if the patient did not have sufficient knowledge on which to pose an intelligent consent, this amounts to no consent and the physician has "assaulted" the patient.

In 1965 Irwin Perr, a lawyer-psychiatrist, discussed the liability of the hospital and psychiatrists in cases of suicide and said, "The basic law is that a hospital owes to its patients a specific duty of care. If it neglects this duty and through the neglect the patient is enabled to commit suicide, the hospital may be liable for its negligence under wrongful death statutes. To determine if there is negligence, it is necessary to establish the degree of care required."[2] This is usually expressed in the following manner: a hospital must exercise such reasonable care and attention for the safety of its patients as their mental and physical conditions may require.

Delegated Legal Responsibilities

What is the responsibility for the resident physician in a large medical center who writes a prescription for a patient being treated by mental health workers, nurses, psychologists, social workers who are part of a treatment team approach? The physician has the ultimate responsibility by virtue of his license to practice medicine and his privilege of writing prescriptions for patients to be sure that no harm comes to the patient no matter who is treating the patient. In a practical sense the resident physician cannot see every patient that comes to the hospital or to the clinic. Often he is rushed and asked to refill a prescription or start a new prescription for a patient who "needs a tranquilizer" or is very depressed and requires antidepressant medication. The resident physician cannot see every patient for whom he writes a prescription in this kind of a setting; yet he does assume the responsibility for medical care of each patient.

What can one do to protect himself against possible damage by virtue of an abreaction to the medication? It seems to me that the best approach would be to assume that the therapist, no matter what his rank, is a part of a "patient complex" of the physician; that is to say, when the resident writes a prescription, he should instruct the therapist regarding the potential dangers of the medication and instruct the patient to report back to the therapist any complications or side reactions that might occur. The therapist then conveys this message, as a physician would if the resident were seeing the patient directly. It is the responsibility then of the resident physician to be sure that any side reactions are reported at the team meetings. Communication becomes the essential feature of such a practice of mass medicine. Perhaps policies ought to be instituted wherein prescriptions are not automatically renewed but the patient's progress is reviewed before such renewal occurs.

From a practical point of view, of course, these measures cannot always occur and one must understand that physicians do take risks in signing prescriptions for patients they do not see, without having time even to instruct the intermediary or the therapist. These risks are real at times and must be considered. However, if one is willing to take a risk for the patient's health, he must also assume the risk of an untoward reaction and possible malpractice suit.

The whole question of the role of the resident physician within a clinic setup or in a mental health setup is an unclear one and guidelines need to be established regarding the responsibility of various members of the treatment team. The author feels the physician should continue to assume the medical responsibility for any patient treated at the clinic. He must, by virtue of his license to practice medicine, take this responsibility and cannot delegate the final care to anyone but himself.

Psychiatry in general or the legal profession has not assumed that "mental illness is a myth" such that social abreactions or adjustment reactions of living do not fall within the medical realm. If and when a mental illness can be reclassified as a social disease or maladjustment syndrome without the medical model to be followed, and without the physician taking the medical responsibility for such illness, then perhaps such responsibility can be delegated to nonmedical personnel. However, at present the law is quite clear, that the physician assumes the responsibility for mental aberrations which may lead to damage to oneself or others. This continues to be classified as mental illness under the medical model and the physician is the ultimate therapist. This conception has led to great interprofessional controversy recently. Nurses are requesting greater professional responsibility and psychologists argue that they are the primary therapists in many cases. As the total care of mentally ill and emotionally disturbed persons expands, the concept of professional responsibility is similarly expanding to include all who care for the patient.

There is a statute of limitations on malpractice cases, the limitation beginning with the time of discovery of the damage. This time limitation may extend from one year in malpractice for torts; i.e. assault and battery or for wrongful death action to two to four years for breach of oral or written contract.

This brief introduction to the subject of malpractice in psychiatry may be supplemented by reading Donald Dawidoff's comprehensive monograph in this series entitled *The Malpractice of Psychiatrists*.[3] A practicing attorney in New York, he presents the legal bases for negligence and malpractice in psychiatry, and includes faulty management of psychoanalysis and psychotherapy, as well as the traditional areas in psychiatry that may lead to a successful malpractice suit.

REFERENCES

1. Bellamy, W. A.: Malpractice risks confronting the psychiatrist: A nationwide fifteen year study of appellate court cases, 1946 to 1961. *Am J Psychiat, 118:*709, 1962.
2. Perr, Irwin: Liability of hospital and psychiatrist in suicide. *Am J Psychiat, 122:*631, 1965.
3. Dawidoff, D. J.: *The Malpractice of Psychiatrists.* Springfield, Thomas, 1973.

Chapter 20

CONFIDENTIALITY AND PRIVILEGE

CONFIDENTIALITY AND PRIVILEGE are two terms which are often confusing to physicians. Confidentiality is an ethical relationship between physician and patient as enunciated in the Hippocratic Oath. "Whatever in connection with my professional practice, or not in connection with it, I see or hear in the life of men which ought not to be spoken of abroad, I will not divulge as reckoning that all such be kept secret." In medicine it is important to keep the confidence of the patient, and particularly in psychiatry it is necessary in order to encourage patients to divulge their innermost secrets. This is especially true in psychoanalysis and in psychoanalytic therapy, wherein the patient must feel completely free to say whatever comes into his mind, no matter how embarrassing, shameful or guilt-producing. One can expect this type of freedom of expression only within a relationship in which absolute confidentiality exists.

The official American Psychiatric Association "Statement of Ethics for Psychiatrists" maintains,

> A physician may not reveal the confidences entrusted to him in the course of medical attendance or the deficiencies he may observe in the character of patients, unless he is required to do so by law or unless it becomes necessary in order to protect the welfare of the individual or of the community. A psychiatrist may release confidential information only with the authorization of the patient or under proper legal compulsion. The continuing duty of the psychiatrist to protect the patient includes fully apprising him of the connotations of waiving the privilege of privacy.... Psychiatrists at times may find it necessary in order to protect the patient or the community from *imminent danger* to reveal confidential information disclosed by the patient.[1]

For the most part, there is no difficulty in maintaining the confidences of one's patients. However, there may be times in which a physician or psychiatrist may be forced to divulge such confidences in a court of law. Ordinarily the patient has a privileged communication with his physician or psychiatrist. This means that the court may not extract this information from the physician if the patient protests, except under special circumstances. In a few states, a special psychotherapist-patient privilege exists in which the psychiatrist is not subject to revealing the information except under the following conditions:

A. The patient is involved in criminal proceedings.
B. There is an emergency situation requiring the physician to act without the consent of the patient.
C. The patient is involved in civil proceedings in which he raises his mental state as an essential factor toward recovering an award or damages.

In these three circumstances there is an automatic waiver of the privilege; i.e. the patient has no control over the testimony of the physician and the psychiatrist is obliged to reveal the information requested.

California recently declared that the psychiatrst need only testify to that information which is relevant to the issue at hand.

The law has traditionally balanced the privilege of the psychiatrist-patient relationship between fostering the confidentiality necessary for optimal therapeutic effect against withholding information which would be necessary for the promotion of social justice.

In 1960 the Group for the Advancement of Psychiatry (GAP) issued a report urging the promotion of privileged communication in the practice of psychiatry. The GAP report concludes,

> The special character of psychiatric treatment . . . requires confidentiality as a *sine qua non* for the successful therapy. . . . The confidential relationship needs to be safeguarded. . . . The psychiatrist best fulfills his professional responsibility to the community by maintaining primary emphasis on problems of treatment. . . . Privilege has been challenged on the grounds that it substantially obstructs justice by withholding evidence. It is our belief that the social value which effective psychiatric treatment has for the community far outweighs

the potential loss of evidence resulting from the withholding of testimony by a psychiatrist about his patient. The absence of privilege, among other results, may obstruct the public need to have unencumbered access to psychiatric treatment sources. Therefore we urge that a patient's communication made to his psychiatrist during the treatment be given the status of unqualified privilege.[2]

Recently, in Pennsylvania, the statute certifying psychologists included a statement granting a privilege equal to that of attorney-client.* Efforts continue to encourage enactment of a general psychotherapist-patient privilege that is more restrictive than the usual physician-patient privilege.

It has been traditionally held that privilege or confidentiality goes out the window in litigation between the parties. Thus, when a patient sues a physician for malpractice he waives his secrecy privilege in relation to the issued involved. The same principle applies in a suit brought by the physicians for the patient's failure to perform his obligation under the contract; i.e. to pay for services rendered. Privilege precludes a third person from calling the physician as a witness against the patient; it is not applicable in suits between physician and patient.

Group Therapy

Questions have arisen regarding confidentiality or privilege in newer forms of therapy, such as group therapy, family therapy or co-therapy. What is the responsibility of the physician for information that may have been leaked by one group member about others in the group?

This is a very important question and occurs quite often as group therapy has recently become a more frequent form of treatment. In beginning a new group and when admitting new members into the group all members should be advised that this is group psychotherapy and that what is divulged within the room should not be transmitted elsewhere. It is necessary to establish a feeling of mutual trust and responsibility, one for the other, and to encourage confidence in the others' revelations.

---

* Senate Bill No. 367, General Assembly, No. 52, March 23, 1973 Effective November 23, 1973, Penna.

On one occasion, when admitting a new patient to a group, one of the old patients recognized the new one and decided that she could not continue in the group because she did not trust the new arrival to keep secret her feelings and her revelations. There is no effective control in group therapy for keeping secrets within the group. Often members of the group will discuss issues generally, and sometimes specifically at home, in order to prove points to their families. One method that works occasionally is to keep the group on a first name basis only, and allow the members to present their names and further identification only if they wish to do so.

With respect to privilege or confidentiality in group psychotherapy, the GAP Report concludes,

> Patients in group therapy develop transferences between themselves, but legally and strictly speaking patients *inter se* do not constitute a physician-patient relationship. Hence it would seem that the medical privilege does not protect against disclosure in court by a member of the group. The privilege exempts only the physician from testifying. It appears necessary to reformulate the medical privilege in view of group therapy, some therapists even predict a time in the near future when patients will be treated primarily in group situations.[2]

Group psychotherapy within prisons has not worked as well as one might hope because of the lack of confidentiality that exists in prisons. Prisoners are frightened of divulging information which could be used against them in the total institution of the prison. The value of the group psychotherapy in prison lies in increasing communication at a safer superficial level and allowing for signs of motivation for improvement when parole is imminent.

Criminal Behavior

How does one handle the problem of a patient in therapy who has admitted to the therapist that he has committed a crime? What obligation does the therapist have to reveal this information and when does he have an obligation not to disclose it? These are difficult questions which reflect the moral and ethical considerations of the therapist. The answer lies in part with the severity of the crime, whether or not someone has been hurt or will be hurt if the information is not disclosed and whether or not disclosing it is helpful or harmful to the patient.

Many psychiatrists would not reveal if a patient admitted smoking marijuana or shoplifting. They see both as reflections of emotional disturbance or mental illness and disclosure would be antitherapeutic, destroying the therapeutic relationship. However, in the instance where someone has been raped, assaulted or killed, the solution is not so simple. Many psychiatrists would unhesitatingly reveal the information to the authorities and others would withhold the information, again for therapeutic reasons.

In some patients, however, it might make more sense and be more helpful if the psychiatrist could convince the patient to turn himself in as a responsible act. If the patient refuses and the psychiatrist feels that his patient represents a danger to society, or to himself, he might, under the doctrine of "emergency situation" reveal the information to a family member or to the police. If the patient will not divulge the information himself, the psychiatrist has a number of alternatives: he may do nothing, he may accompany the patient to the proper authorities or he may indicate to the patient that he will have to tell the patient's relatives (father, mother, spouse) about this behavior and encourage the responsible family member to take the patient to the police.

There are many levels of handling such information without either keeping it secret or immediately divulging it. For example, one has to consider whether or not the patient is indulging in fantasy; is he lying or testing the psychiatrist? One should not jump in without being sure of his information.

Adolescents

What is the extent of the confidential relationship between an adolescent and his psychiatrist, and when must the psychiatrist reveal information to the youngster's parents? In examining any adolescent for the first time, the presence of a parent is helpful. Following the initial examination a discussion of the evaluation with the parents and child should take place. The parents should know that there will be times during the course of therapy when they will not be told things that the patient has said. The parent is encouraged to call and reveal any information about his youngster that will help make treatment more effective. The author usually does not divulge to parents if their youngsters say they have smoked marijuana or that they are having sexual intercourse or that they have a venereal disease or they are pregnant. The youngsters are encouraged to tell their parents themselves and to try and deal with the consequences as realistically as possible. Thus, *limits of confidentially* are set at the beginning of therapy.

When told properly, parents can accept and appreciate the candor of the psychiatrist and will remember the statements subsequently when they are seeking information and are denied satisfaction. The youngster usually appreciates the honesty and integrity of the psychiatrist, and begins to trust him after many, many tests, to see whether or not he meant what he said.

Probation and Parole

In treating patients who are on probation or parole, a letter is often requested on a quarterly or semiannual basis to the probation office, indicating the progress of the patient. Assuming no untoward reaction or legal difficulty the patient has had, it is not necessary to divulge to the probation officer the intimacies shared by the patient. What the author usually puts into such a report is that the patient either has attended regularly or he has not, that he has been responsible financially for the therapy and that he seems to be making progress or not, as the case may be. Often these letters are required to be sent to judges who are interested in their people on probation. Whenever letters are sent to anyone, even to another physician about a patient, the patient is required to sign an authorized form to release the information. This should be kept on file in the event the patient is unhappy about what was said to another agency or physician.

Records and Subpoenaes

Some psychiatrists keep no records at all, others keep only attendance and financial records, and some keep extensive records in a hidden file which is never available to anyone else, not even to subpoena. They keep a separate file with shorter notes and no intimate details. It can be dangerous to patients and others if the intimate details of a therapeutic relationship fall into the wrong hands.

In one case a woman had presented her unconscious utterings of homosexual fantasies that the analyst jotted down on his note pad. When a divorce action ensued, her husband's attorney subpoenaed the records of the psychiatrist in order to prove that she was mentally unbalanced. The psychiatrist foolishly allowed his notes, rather than a formal record, to leave his office. The subpoena was issued by the judge and the notes were to go only to the judge in the strictest confidence. The judge shared the information with the lawyer for the husband, who foolishly showed them to the husband, who became enraged and immediately proceeded to his wife's residence and severely beat her, necessitating her hospitalization.

Granted, this is a unique and rare case, but it serves to illustrate the extent of damage that can ensue from the misuse of psychiatric information. Personal intimate notes of this type are never appropriate for court action and should never be allowed to leave the psychiatrist's office. What the court needs to know can be given in a summary statement, including diagnosis, prognosis, progress of the patient and specific difficulties encountered in the illness. The type of medication, response to medication, side effects, etc. are also important but unconscious utterings, unless they are understood within the comprehensive context of the patient's illness, are not appropriate for other than the psychiatrist's office.

Insurance and Psychiatry

Insurance companies are one of the "third parties" which require information about patients from time to time. The psychiatrist is well advised to have a signed release of information by the patient before releasing any information to anyone. The patient should be informed about requests for information. Often the patient can be told exactly what will be included in the statement. What patients may sign at some earlier time may not always be in their best interest and they may not want certain information divulged. They have a right to know what the psychiatrist will say about them and to whom.

In summary, the psychiatrist should maintain a strict confidential relationship with his patient and should never divulge information without the consent of the patient. The exceptions are emergencies, criminal actions and court-ordered statements. There are borderline cases in which the patient may need to be encouraged to divulge the information himself or it may become an urgent or emergent situation. If the psychiatrist divulges information without the consent of the patient, and the patient suffers damage because of this revelation, the psychiatrist may be subject to a malpractice suit. The psychiatrist has a duty to maintain confidence; divulgence of secrets is a dereliction of this duty. If it results directly in damage to the patient it satisfies the necessary criteria for negligence or malpractice. The psychiatrist must protect himself and his family against such malpractice suits by keeping his patients' confidences to himself and not being careless in social situations.

Anyone working for psychiatrists, such as a secretary, receptionist or associate, is considered by law to be his agent. If confidence is breached through agents of the psychiatrist, the psychiatrist is held responsible and potentially liable. The psychiatrist must brief his employees and associates about the need for strict confidentiality because it is his professional standing which could be jeopardized by their loose tongues.

Wahl[3] has written on the treatment of the rich, famous and influential, and indicates that psychiatrists are more apt to "name-drop" this type of patient in part to satisfy their own ego demands and to show that they are "good therapists" to treat such a person. This careless behavior could be dangerous in that it may damage the patient and the psychiatrist may be found negligent. It is safest to never acknowledge that a person is one's patient. The psychiatrist should be extremely careful in revealing to anyone who his patient is, or anything about his patient until he is certain of the identity of the person requesting the information and the purpose to which the information will be put.

This occurred in the case of a woman who had become acutely schizophrenic, was hospitalized with delusions of grandeur and persecution, and delusions of reference that radio commentators were directly addressing her, and she would follow their orders. When in the hospital, and psychotic, her husband asked about her condition. He was told that her condition was diagnosed as an acute schizophrenic reaction, paranoid type and that with proper treatment and medication her prognosis was favorable for this occurrence, but that it was likely to recur under stress in the future. After several weeks she improved considerably and upon improvement, she decided that she wished to leave her husband and take her four-year-old daughter with her. Her husband construed this wish of hers to be a product of her mental illness and decided to contest her divorce and her custody of their child.

Several weeks after the patient was discharged from the hospital a letter from an attorney, requesting information about the patient was received. He had enclosed a signed "authorized" release of information form signed by her husband. Obviously the husband wished to use the information against his wife. It would not be proper to give him this information in writing without the consent of his wife, who, when asked, refused.

This case raises the issue of informed consent in psychiatry and specifically in forensic psychiatry. Informed consent is the basic concept involved in release of psychiatric information. In medicine generally a patient needs to know the nature of any medical or surgical procedure to be performed upon him, the risks and the chances for success before his consent can be considered "informed." In psychiatry, the examination is the procedure. Whenever and wherever possible, the patient must know the purposes of such an examination, to whom the findings will be made available, and what consequences may befall him as a result of his revelations.

In both civil and criminal law, the authorization for release of information can be faulty, incomplete or fraudulent. The psychiatrist should be wary not only of the lack of informed consent but of inappropriate use of his professional standing.

In civil law informed consent would appear to be a relatively straightforward matter but sometimes the issue can become confused. In cases of domestic relations, especially when child custody or visitation rights are involved, full knowledge of the purpose of the examination and how the psychiatric report will be used is essential for all parties concerned.

Commitment procedures represent another large area in which the purpose of psychiatric examinations must be clear to the patient. A housewife sued a psychiatrist for malpractice not long ago, alleging that he had treated her against her will while she was temporarily hospitalized in a private mental institution following a court order. At issue was what had occurred when the psychiatrist made a house call to the plaintiff's home and introduced himself as a physician. The psychiatrist admitted that he had never met the housewife or her husband before making the visit. He stated that he had been called by the husband to examine the woman.

The psychiatrist allegedly told the housewife that he had come to examine her husband and to evaluate his back problem. Apparently he never told the woman he was a psychiatrist. On another occasion when the wife spoke with the psychiatrist after a quarrel in the household, he again did not tell her his professional specialty.

Within that month, the woman's suit charged, the psychiatrist together with another physician "at the request of the plaintiff's husband, and without the authorization, knowledge or consent of plaintiff, signed a sworn statement certifying that they had examined her and found her to be mentally ill." What had followed, of course, was her involuntary commitment to the private mental hospital where she was forced to accept treatment she did not want.

What concerns me here is the deception of the psychiatrist in examining the patient without telling her who he was or why he was there. As a result, she was not properly informed to give consent to the doctor's examination and his questioning of her.

Obtaining informed consent prior to determination of competency is a complex issue. Can an incompetent person understand the nature of the examination and the purposes to which the report will be put? Does he have the capacity to give informed consent? Other significant issues include the patient's right to refuse the examination and the ethical and legal responsibilities of psychiatric reporting of sensitive information.

Psychological testing for employment purposes or psychiatric examinations in industry represent another area in which the concepts of informed consent is relevant. Virtually any probe into the unconscious by a physician who wears two hats, the medical and the administrative, may be fraught with the possibility of breach of confidentiality. People must have the right to refuse such probes. In order to do so, they must be fully informed about the nature of the investigation.

In criminal law informed consent also affects disclosure of information. A defendant may be examined prior to trial or before sentence, either by a defense psychiatrist, a prosecution psychiatrist, or a court-appointed one. A prison psychiatrist may examine an inmate for possible release on parole. A probationer may be examined to determine whether he is "safe" to remain unconfined. In each case the defendant must know the nature of the examination, whom the psychiatrist represents and to what purpose the information he reveals will be put.

Several years ago, a man awaiting trial was befriended by a psychiatrist posing as a fellow inmate in a county jail. Actually, this was a ploy by the psychiatrist to obtain a confession from the defendant. In the subsequent trial, the psychiatrist's testimony of statements made by the defendant was admitted into evidence. The man was found guilty. On appeal, the psychiatrist's trial testimony was rejected. The psychiatrist was chastized by the court for resorting to such trickery. He had obtained the information without the informed consent of the defendant.

A thirty-year-old defendant was examined by a court clinic

psychiatrist to determine his competency to stand trial. At the time of the examination, no mention was made of other uses to which the report would be put. Neither was any effort made to determine the defendant's state of mind at the time of the crime for determination of criminal responsibility. During the trial, however, the district attorney called the examining psychiatrist to testify, not to competency, but to the question of criminal responsibility.

Ideally, the psychiatrist should have testified that he was in no position to make such a determination since he did not examine the defendant with that in mind, nor did he tell the defendant that he was going to examine him for that purpose. Instead, the psychiatrist indicated that in his opinion the defendant was not insane under the M'Naghten Rule at the time of the offense.

As an impartial professional, the psychiatrist should not find the principle of informed consent a problem. In the following instance the author was asked to examine a defendant for the court, another for the public defender's office and the other for the prosecutor. To each of the interviewees it was carefully explained who the author was, who called for the interview, what the consequences of their verbalizations would be, to whom my report would be sent and what it might mean to them in terms of their case. The suspect was told if the examination was for the prosecutor, just whom the interviewer represented and that he should be guided by that information before he spoke. He was more than willing to talk; he knew that if he got a "clean bill of health"—determination on my part that he was not seriously emotionally ill—the charges would be diminished and he would not be sent to prison.

On another occasion, a prosecutor asked the author to examine a prison inmate in the company of another psychiatrist and a psychologist. These two professionals were eminently qualified and experienced, having worked in court clinic facilities for years. When we arrived at the prison, the defendant's lawyer was present. The defendant very clearly and deliberately stated that he was present out of respect for our position but that he respectfully declined to answer any questions we might ask.

The psychologist immediately "threatened" the man by saying

that if he did not speak to us it would be presumed that he was mentally ill and that he would likely be sent to the state hospital for the criminally insane, where he might spend many years awaiting trial. The author chastized the psychologist for his inappropriate comment and his threat to the patient/defendant.

The defendant was then informed that no such steps would necessarily occur and that he certainly had the right to have a psychiatrist called in by his own lawyer to examine him for the purposes of competency and criminal responsibility. The defendant was told that he had every right to refuse to talk with us and that it would not necessarily be harmful to him if he refused. Finally he was told that no presumptions about his mental illness or state of mind would be made if he did not talk with us.

We had come to the prison and had met with the man, and he respectfully declined to discuss the matter at hand with us. To have forced an interview under the threat of pretrial commitment would have been ethically, if not legally, indefensible. It is precisely this kind of abuse of power by psychiatrists that we must diligently guard against.

The patient, no matter who he is, has a fundamental right to know the identity of the psychiatrist or psychologist who is questioning him. He has a right to know whom that professional represents and the purpose of the interview or examination. If he is given this information, his consent to be examined or interviewed truly will be an informed one. Further, he should have the right to refuse to cooperate if he so chooses. If the psychiatrist understands these concepts and adheres to them, he will be practicing according to the highest standards of our profession.

REFERENCES

1. Statement of ethics for psychiatrists. *Am J Psychiat, 130*:9, 1063, 1973.
2. Group for the Advancement of Psychiatry (GAP) Report #45 *Confidentiality and Privileged Communication in the Practice of Psychiatry.* New York, June, 1960.
3. Wahl, C. W.: Psychoanalysis of the rich, the famous and the influential. Presented at the annual meeting of the APA, Washington, D.C., May, 1971.

GLOSSARY

ABREACTION: That form of reaction that a person experiences when recalling or reliving an earlier traumatic situation. This is usually done under hypnosis, narcoanalysis or psychotherapy. Suddenly the individual is confronted with an earlier trauma which he has repressed and abreacts; i.e. reacts emotionally to the emergence of the conflict which has been kept alive through repression.

ACT OUT: A person is said to act out his emotional conflicts if he externalizes them rather than internalizing them in a psychoneurotic way. Acting out is a behavior manifestation of emotional conflicts and is most often seen as a symptom of sociopathic or antisocial personality.

ACUTE: Acute is a short-lived intense reaction as opposed to chronic, which is long-term. The prognosis or outlook for an acute reaction is usually quite good.

ACUTE BRAIN SYNDROME: Refers to a category of organic brain illness which is acute, short-lived and quite intense. It is usually associated with some other physical illness which affects the brain.

ADJUSTMENT: The organism's or individual's ability to cope with various stresses or environmental situations. There is also an adjustment reaction of adolescence or childhood which means that an individual has difficulty in coping or adjusting to his environment.

AFFECT: Feeling tone. Usually refers to anxiety, depression or mania.

Material contained in this Glossary is reprinted with permission from the volume on *Psychic Injuries,* contained in the series, *Courtroom Medicine,* © 1975, Matthew Bender & Co.

AFFECTIVE REACTION: A reaction in the individual, usually of an extreme nature, which may be pathological either of extreme depression or anxiety.

AGGRESSION: The normal aggressive tendencies of the individual, not necessarily hostility. All organisms possess some form of aggressiveness or aggression in order to survive.

AGORAPHOBIA: A fear of open spaces.

ALCOHOLISM: The condition of being an alcoholic; i.e. addicted to alcohol. Alcoholics are unable to stop drinking as long as alcohol is present unless they pass out or otherwise are kept from the alcohol.

AMBIVALENCE: The feeling of confusion or mixed feelings about a certain subject or event. A person may be ambivalent if he has both positive and negative feelings about someone or something.

AMNESIA: The forgetting at a later time of events from a previous time which one ordinarily should have or would have remembered. The amnesia may be caused by emotional trauma, emotional illness, chemical interference (alcohol or drugs) or physical trauma, a blow to the head.

ANALYST: Another name for a psychoanalyst who is a psychiatrist who has completed several years of advanced training in psychoanalysis and has had adequate supervision of control cases.

ANOREXIA: The inability to eat, usually on an emotional basis. Anorexia nervosa is a psychotic illness usually found in adolescent females who die unless they are tube fed or treated with intensive measures.

ANTISOCIAL PERSONALITY: A diagnostic category of personality disorder manifested primarily by antisocial behavior, inability to learn from previous experiences and lack of clear conscience.

ANXIETY: That form of emotion which indicates heightened tension or a feeling of "unease."

ASTHENIA: A physical weakness with emotional manifestations.

AUTISM: Most often seen in children who are called "autistic" or early psychotic. The child or individual who is autistic deals with his own fantasies and internal conflicts in an idiosyncratic way, not usually related to external reality.

BENIGN: Benign as opposed to malignant means a nonprogressive, nonlife-threatening illness and one which may be self-limited.

BRAIN: The physical substance or tissue of the brain as opposed to the mind.

CATATONIC: The type of schizophrenic who shows limited movement, usually is unable to move, is silent and nonresponsive. He shows waxy flexibility.

CATHARSIS: The flow of emotion that often is quite therapeutic. A person may have an emotional catharsis if he spills out the feelings and anxieties that he has held inside.

CATHEXIS: The involvement of an individual emotionally with others. That is, an individual is said to have a cathexis or an investment or interest in someone or something else.

CEREBRUM: Refers to the major hemispheres of the brain. *Cerebral* often means thinking or function of intelligence, but technically is a function of the brain.

CHARACTER: A type of personality; in psychiatry is usually referred to as a character disorder or personality disorder.

CHARACTER TRAITS: Those traits related to an individual's specific character. A person may have an hysterical trait; that is, handling his anxiety by repression or denial. He may have obsessive-compulsive traits, which mean that he is orderly and neat and tends to organize factors around him in order to regulate or control his anxiety.

CHRONIC: Means long-standing, describing an illness whose prognosis usually is not good especially if untreated.

CHRONIC BRAIN SYNDROME: See acute brain syndrome. Is also an organic illness of the brain which is chronic and usually related to some other physical disease which involves the brain.

CLAUSTROPHOBIA: A specific fear of closed-in places such as elevators, crowded buses or airplanes.

CLINICAL: Refers to the psychiatric examination or the clinical examination, as opposed to a paper-and-pencil psychological test evaluation.

CLINICAL SYMPTOMS: Those observed by the individual and reportable to his doctor.

COMA: A person is said to be in coma if he is unconscious and nonresponsive. The cause of the coma may be illness, trauma or infection.

COMPLEX: A symptom complex may be a group of symptoms which form an illness or a syndrome. A person may also have a complex; i.e. a specific reaction to people or things about him.

COMPULSIVE DISORDER: A disorder characterized by compulsive behavior such as hand-washing or knob-touching or counting or dressing rituals.

CONATION: Feeling tone as opposed to cognition, which refers to intellectualization.

CONCUSSION: An injury to the brain manifested primarily by bruising as opposed to tearing. It is a bump of the brain against the hard bony skull, usually by a blow to the head.

CONFABULATION: The making up of stories or situations to fill in gaps in one's background or history. One lies or confabulates especially if he does not remember and cannot tolerate the fact that he doesn't remember. Usually seen in elderly people and those with brain damage.

CONSCIOUS: Awake, alert. It is also that part of the mind, as described by Freud, that is aware of external surroundings.

CONTUSION: A laceration of the brain substance.

CONVERSION REACTION: That form of psychoneurotic reaction of the hysterical type in which emotional conflicts are converted into physical symptoms. For example, the fear of flying in battle in a pilot may be converted into a paralysis of his hand in order to save face and justify his not flying. The primary gain is the avoidance of the fear of dying in the aircraft and the secondary gain may be the rest he obtains from the illness or satisfaction of dependency needs.

DEFENSE MECHANISM: All individuals and organisms have defense mechanisms whereby they protect themselves and handle external attacks and internal anxiety states. Examples of defense mechanisms are rationalization, introjection, compensation and denial. They are ego functions.

DELIRIUM: A specific state of anxiety and agitation usually caused by chemical means such as alcohol or drugs in which an individual is out of touch with reality, psychotic. Specifically, *delirium tremens* is a delirium caused by withdrawal of alcohol in which the individual shakes profusely and may have hallucinations and delusions.

DELUSION: A misperception of reality by thinking. One may have a delusion of grandiosity, of persecution or a delusion of self-reference. All may be involved in a paranoid illness.

DEMENTIA: A serious psychotic state of illness of the mind or emotions. Specifically, *dementia praecox,* the original name for schizophrenia, an illness that begins in the young.

DENIAL: A defense mechanism characterized by either a conscious or unconscious denial of anxiety and conflicts.

DEPENDENCY: Usually refers to a characterological or personality disorder in which an individual is overly dependent on others.

DEPERSONALIZATION: A feeling that an individual may have that is usually pathological, but not necessarily so, where he feels that he is not personally involved in his external surroundings. He feels apart from a situation in which he is involved.

DEPRESSION: An affective reaction of low mood. There are all forms of depression which may be characterized from a "blue mood" to a psychotic depression. Basically the difference is one of degree rather than quality. All of us have been blue or depressed when things don't go right. We talk about feeling blue if the stock market is down or if the day is rainy and a picnic was planned. This is mostly disappointment. Beyond disappointment is depression which may be characterized by difficulty in eating or sleeping, some anxiety or agitation, feeling of uneasiness. As the depression becomes deeper a person shows psychomotor retardation (inability to move freely or easily about), wanting to stay in bed, social isolation, lack of energy to become involved in anything around him, insomnia, anorexia (lack of appetite) and eventually feelings of hopelessness, helplessness, and suicidal ideation, gestures and attempts.

DISORIENTATION: An individual who is not oriented in three spheres, person, place and time. Does he know who he is, where he is and the approximate date? Disorientation is quite important in the evaluation of mental illness and is usually found in people who are organically ill or severely functionally ill.

DISPLACEMENT: A mechanism of defense by which an individual displaces characteristics of one situation or object onto another in order to help ward off anxiety.

DISSOCIATIVE REACTION: Form of psychoneurotic reaction, hysterical type, in which there is a dissociation between feeling tone and thoughts. A person may dissociate (separate) his affect, his feelings from external reality and act in an altered state of consciousness. One of the extensions or extremes of a dissociative reaction is the *fugue state*, in which an individual assumes another personality or multiple personality, as exemplied in *The Three Faces of Eve*.

DRIVE: The primary urges or drives of the organism that each individual has.

DYNAMIC: Also *psychodynamic*. Factors involved in illness or aberrant behavior.

DYSSOCIAL REACTION: A diagnostic category of a personality disorder, usually manifested by antisocial behavior which is a part of a cultural norm. That is, an individual who commits antisocial acts that are approved by the smaller society to which he belongs would be called dyssocial rather than antisocial.

EGO: That part of the triad of id, ego, superego which refers to the judgmental functions of the individual, the mediator between the urges of the id and the conscience of the superego.

EGO IDEAL: The model found in the superego that the individual wishes to be like. In some cases in which the superego or the conscience is extremely harsh, the ego ideal is punitive, leading to difficulties in behavior. If the ego ideal is excessively light an individual may have difficulty following rules.

ELECTROENCEPHALOGRAM: A brain wave tracing. This is obtained by use of needles or electrodes on the scalp which pick up the electrical impulses of the brain. These are used primarily to detect aberrations of electrical conduction as found in seizure disorders, growths or tumors in the brain or other cerebral changes.

ENURESIS: Bed-wetting beyond the usually expected age of bladder control (after the age of 5 or 6).

EPILEPSY: A condition of the brain which results in seizures. These seizures may be of three types. (a) Grand mal seizure, which is the loss of consciousness with typical tongue biting and gagging and loss of continence. (b) Petit mal is the smaller seizure usually seen in younger individuals which may be manifested only by momentary loss of consciousness without falling. There is no incontinence, no tonic and clonic phases but merely a break with the continuity of time. (c) Psychomotor seizures usually originate in the temporal lobe of the brain and may be manifested primarily by aberrant behavior.

ETIOLOGY: Cause, especially of an illness.

EUPHORIA: A heightened feeling of affect, that is, an excessively high feeling on the part of an individual of a positive nature but which is extreme and often pathological.

EXHIBITIONIST: An individual who exposes his genitals in public but more generally may mean an individual who is a "show-off" or one who has little modesty.

Fellatio: Oral sexual act committed on the male.

Filicide: The killing of one's child.

Forensic psychiatry: That branch of psychiatry dealing with mental and emotional illness related to legal situations, both civil and criminal.

Fugue: An extreme form of psychoneurotic hysterical reaction, dissociative type, in which there is a dissociation between reality and affect. Thus in a fugue state a person may be living one life and has repressed and denied the existence of another former life. These are extreme forms of multiple personality and are quite rare.

Functional: Used to denote an illness which is not related to an organic or physical illness but is primarily emotional or mental.

Ganzer Syndrome: A specific illness found in individuals in prisons or under serious stress which is characterized by an exaggeration of bizarre symptoms and may be a psychosis. Some people feel that the Ganzer Syndrome reflects a conscious exaggeration or malingering rather than a psychotic state.

Globus hystericus: A symptom of psychoneurotic hysterical reaction in which the individual experiences a ball or a globule in his throat on swallowing. It is a choking sensation, especially prominent during breathing and talking and more significantly during excessive anxiety. It may follow a physical trauma.

Gross stress reaction: The reaction by an individual under acute stress and characterized by a gross rather than specific reaction in any particular organ.

Hallucination: A misperception, either visually or audibly by an individual when no particular stimuli are present. That is, a person may hear voices when no one is present around him and the voices may talk about him or to him. Or, he may see visions which are not present; e.g. the so-called "pink elephants" of the toxic alcoholic. The visual hallucinations are more commonly found in organic illness and the auditory hallucinations in a functional illness.

HOMOSEXUALITY: The preference of an individual sexually for a member of his own sex.

HYPOCHONDRIASIS: A condition of an individual who has a fear that he is ill in many ways. He will characterize himself as having difficulties in all areas of his body and mind, and often feels that his functions are impaired and sometimes that his body is deteriorating.

HYSTERIA: A confusing word in psychiatry that may mean a number of things. First, hysteria is used by the layman to denote *panic;* i.e. a person is hysterical, crying excessively without control and in a state of near panic. Hysteria may refer to a *personality disorder* characterized by repression and denial; i.e. an individual who may be coquettish, usually a woman who is flirtatious and has little emotional depth. Hysterical *neurosis* refers to the two types of illness, one characterized by *conversion* symptoms—conversion of emotional conflicts into physical symptoms, with evidence of secondary gain and no organic pathology. Secondly, in the *dissociative reaction* the emotions are dissociated from the thought processes. Finally, hysteria may refer to the *defense mechanisms* of repression and denial and superficiality of emotions. In the original Greek it means "wandering uterus" and usually has been used in reference to women.

IATROGENIC: Caused by the medical profession. A symptom or a condition may be iatrogenic because its etiology was due to a procedure or a statement made by a physician.

ID: That part of the psychic structure outlined by Freud (id, ego, superego) which houses the instincts and primary urges.

IDENTIFICATION: A defense mechanism characterized by the identification of characteristics of an older, aggressive individual. One may identify with someone else in order to protect himself from anticipated threatened or real harm by the other individual.

IMPOTENCE: Usually refers to a feeling of powerlessness and may be used as emotional impotence, but more specifically sexual impotence, in which a male is unable to obtain an erection. Partial impotence refers to the inability of the male to maintain an erection.

INSANITY: A legal concept that refers to conditions of individuals who have mental illness because of which they are unable to meet certain legal criteria. In the M'Naghten Rule, for example, insanity refers to the inability to know the nature and quality of one's act at the time one committed it, or if he did, that he did not know that it was wrong. Other tests of criminal responsibility also test for insanity at the time of a particular act.

INSIGHT: Used by psychiatrists to denote a person's ability to recognize his own internal needs and goals, and reasons for his behavior and his symptoms.

INSOMNIA: An inability to sleep, usually found in depressed individuals or those who are extremely anxious.

INTROJECTION: Another defense mechanism characterized by the internalization of certain features or characteristics of individuals in one's life history. One will introject, for example, qualities of one's father.

INVOLUTION: Used with depression and refers to the depressive symptoms associated with menopause.

INVOLUTIONAL MELANCHOLIA: A psychotic depressive illness which occurs about the time of menopause.

IQ (INTELLIGENCE QUOTIENT): Is a measure of a person's intelligence, usually determined by one of several standard tests. The average IQ is 100.

ISOLATION: Defense mechanism which is used in order to isolate out certain feelings or separate them from others.

KLEPTOMANIA: A category of emotional illness which refers to the individual who is unable to keep from stealing small objects, not because he needs them, but because they are symbolically significant for maintaining or resolving specific emotional conflicts.

LA BELLE INDIFFERENCE: This French phrase characterizes an individual who has a conversion reaction and seems to have little concern about the symptoms he describes.

LATENT: Pending, underlying or potential. When one speaks of a latent schizophrenia, he speaks of an individual who, under proper stress, could become schizophrenic or psychotic.

LIBIDO: A positive emotional involvement, usually of love. One has libidinal ties or shows a libido for someone else. Libido is an emotional investment of a strong positive nature.

MALIGNANT: A term reserved for illnesses that are life-threatening and will progress unless effectively treated.

MALINGERING: The malingerer is one who exaggerates with conscious deception the symptoms that he claims. Malingering may be seen most commonly in those people who have been injured either in a working situation or in an automobile accident. The primary gain for the malingerer is to receive the compensation or the money from being ill. Examples of the classical malingerer are the following: (a) One who claims he is unable because of a weakness or a pain in his back to lift boxes or materials required of him at work and then is seen by a detective, changing a flat tire on his car without difficulty. (b) The woman who claims she is unable to walk without her cane and comes limping into court to complain about her difficulties following her accident and then is seen on movies taken by a private investigator walking very briskly and sprightly without the use of the cane.

MANIA: A hyperactive condition in an individual who speaks rapidly. Hypomania is a bit less than the extreme psychotic condition of mania. The mania may be part of a manic-depressive psychosis which is an alternation between mania and depression, both of which are psychotic and require treatment, often hospitalization. The depressive aspect of manic-depression has been treated effectively with electroshock therapy. More recently, lithium carbonate has been used in the treatment of the manic episodes and prevents the depth of reaction of the manic-depressive illness.

MASOCHISM: Generally means self-hurting; a person who enjoys being hurt by others. He is then spoken of as having a masochistic personality. Specifically, however, masochism refers to the sexual deviation of enjoying pain and obtaining sexual gratification from being physically hurt.

MENTAL DEFECTIVE: A name given to the intellectually retarded. It replaces the earlier categorization of idiot, imbecile and moron.

MIND: The mental functioning of the individual.

MORBIDITY: Refers to illness or sickness, or symptoms of pain or discomfort associated with an illness.

NARCISSISM: That condition which is often referred to as self-love or attention-getting. A person who finds satisfaction or gratification in his own image is said to be narcissistic.

NARCOANALYSIS: The analysis of an individual under the effect of drugs or narcotics. Specifically, what is used is sodium pentothal or sodium amytal. The drugs are used to help the individual become more aware of underlying thoughts, feelings or previous events that have been repressed.

NARCOLEPSY: The condition of sleepwalking; i.e. under the influence of sleep, one has certain reactions such as walking or performing tasks.

NEOLOGISM: A new word made up by an individual who is psychotic and is often seen in schizophrenia. An example of a neologism may be "parahydropharmacognapsycho" or a simple one of combining two words into one such as "television" and "radio" and calling it "radavision" or mispronouncing a word such as "television" and calling it "tvision."

NEURASTHENIA: An emotional or nervous weakness, a condition described in the late 1800's, characterized by anxiety, emotional weakness, inability to function effectively.

NEUROSIS OR PSYCHONEUROSIS: A moderate mental and emotional illness in which an individual shows symptoms which alter his effectiveness and his ability to work or live comfortably but which do not deprive him of his contact with reality.

OBJECT RELATIONS: Those individuals who are significant in a person's life and upon whom he is dependent and toward whom he shows specific conflicts.

OBSESSION: A rumination, a thought organization about a certain subject. A person may be obsessive about his work and continuously think about it and ways to improve it. Usually however, obsession is a rumination which is not progressive and the obsessive individual exerts much emotional energy without constructive results.

OBSESSIVE-COMPULSIVE REACTION: That psychoneurotic reaction a person experiences who continues to ruminate in his thoughts about a certain subject and acts in a compulsive fashion. The obsession is the thinking and the compulsion is behaving. The person who is obsessive-compulsive may go through a series of rituals designed to protect him from anxiety but which eventually paralyze him from functioning effectively.

OEDIPUS COMPLEX: That emotional complex described by Sigmund Freud which originates in the individual, usually the male, at about the age of four or five. It is characterized by the young boy having libidinal affection for his mother and murderous impulses toward his father. Freud saw this as a universal complex which needed to be resolved in order for the individual to progress to a genital form of functioning which he considered to be mature. The word comes from the early Greek tragedy of Oedipus Rex, who was found to have married his mother and killed his father.

ORAL STAGE: There are different stages of psychosexual development as described by Freud and these stages include the oral, anal, phallic, latent, and genital. Basically the oral stage lasts from birth until 1½ yr of age and is characterized by oral gratification. Later manifestations of this stage in the personality include excessive dependency. There may be signs such as smoking or drinking excessively or drug-taking which people have ascribed to an oral personality.

The *phallic stage* lasts from the age of three until about six or seven and includes the Oedipal Complex within it. The phallic stage is characterized by primary gratification in the individual with his phallus. There we see young boys who expose themselves and exhibit themselves and begin to touch their penis in order to obtain pleasant sensations. Later manifestations of the phallic phase include those individuals who are highly pushy and aggressive and some of the exhibitionists.

The *latent stage* is a phase of psychosexual dormancy from the age of about seven to puberty, eleven or twelve. This is the stage of greatest learning during which the individual has put aside some of the conflicts which have occupied his mind for the first six or seven years of his life and is able to utilize the latent phase for constructive learning procedures.

The *genital stage* which begins about the time of puberty and goes through adolescence isn't really mature or complete until after early adulthood. There is a prolonged maturation with the use of genital functioning that is not a phallic or an ineffective pushing or exhibitionism, but a true concern and consideration for other people as well as one's own gratification.

ORGANIC: Refers to physical structural illness rather than functional or emotional illness.

PARANOIA: A condition characterized by projection of one's feelings onto others and delusions of reference whether persecutory or grandiose. It is usually a psychotic illness and may be associated with schizophrenia or may be a pure paranoia without the disintegration of the personality.

PASSIVE-AGGRESSIVE: A personality disorder which is often used as a "waste-basket" diagnosis since so many people show passive-aggressive traits. If there are no other outstanding symptoms, and yet a person shows a passivity in which he is able to obtain gratification, this may be seen as an aggressive phenomenon which is handled in a passive manner. Often these people are annoying to others and difficult to get along with because they take so much from others and give so little of their own.

PATHOLOGICAL LIAR: An individual who tells lies and often does not know that he is telling lies and is unable to control himself.

PERSONALITY: The functioning of the individual, the characterization of him in terms of his thoughts, feelings and behavior.

PHOBIA: A specific psychoneurotic condition which refers to intense fear of a specified nature. For example, an acrophobia—fear of high places.

POTENTIATE: One drug potentiates the action of another if it increases its effect. If the drugs are additive in effect they potentiate each other.

PRECONSCIOUS: Is that part of the mind which is between the conscious and the unconscious. It is from the preconscious that one notes "slips of the tongue" and other events which are not completely conscious. Material in the preconscious is available without use of dream interpretation, free association or narcoanalysis.

PREMORBID: Refers to the personality of the individual prior to the illness or the trauma which he experiences.

PRIMARY PROCESS: The early thinking procedures which occur in children and are illogical but related to emotional and immature goal orientation.

SECONDARY PROCESS: The logical, goal-directed thought processes which most adults possess. The primary process thinking occurs primarily in schizophrenics and severely emotionally deprived individuals.

PRODROMATA: Are those symptoms that one experiences prior to an episode such as a seizure.

PROGNOSIS: The outlook or future prediction of how the individual will recover from his illness. Whether he will be well again or maintain his state of illness, is the prediction or prognosis.

PROJECTION: The defense mechanism of projecting blame or conflicts onto others that one has for himself. He is ashamed or embarrassed of his feelings and is unable to accept them as his own; thus, they are projected onto others. It isn't that "I don't like you" but it's that "you don't like me" and that's why "we don't get along." This is one of the symptoms often found in paranoid individuals.

PSYCHE: Another name for the mind or the personality and often is used quite loosely in the vernacular.

PSYCHIATRIST: A physician who has specialized in the medical speciality of psychiatry and is able to evaluate individuals from the clinical point of view, conduct psychotherapy and also write prescriptions for medication.

PSYCHOANALYSIS: A specific form of evaluating and treating and studying an individual. It is fairly ritualized form in which the analysand (patient) lies on a couch with the psychoanalyst behind him and beyond his view. The sessions last for forty-five to fifty minutes and occur four or five days per week, usually for four or five years. The primary tools in psychoanalysis are free association and analysis of the transference relationship the patient establishes toward the analyst during different stages of the analytic process.

PSYCHODYNAMIC: Refers to those factors involved in an illness which may be evaluated by use of Freudian or psychoanalytic techniques. They are the psychodynamic factors relating to conflicts and relationships among significant people in a person's life.

PSYCHOGENIC: Factors that influence an individual or his illness are referred to as psychogenic factors if they originate in the "psyche" or mind.

PSYCHOLOGIST: An individual who is trained in psychology, usually has a Ph.D. and is able and trained to administer psychological tests for evaluation and diagnosis and also to treat individuals with psychotherapy.

PSYCYOPATH: An old name for the sociopath or the antisocial personality. It is an individual who acts out his internal conflicts and often gets into difficulty with the law, does not learn by previous mistakes and has little or no conscience.

PSYCHOPATHOLOGY: Refers to the illness a person has of a psychic or emotional nature. It does not necessarily refer to a psychopath but is a more general term that means emotional illness.

PSYCHOPHYSIOLOGICAL: Also refers to a psychosomatic and is almost a synonym for it. A symptom may be psychophysiologic if there are physiological problems within the individual such as constipation, diarrhea, excessive flow of hormones due to glandular imbalance.

PSYCHOSIS: A major mental illness in which the individual loses touch with reality.

PSYCHOSOMATIC: Refers to symptoms that appear to be physical in nature but are related to emotional conflicts and caused by emotional difficulties rather than by actual organic tissue pathology.

PSYCHOSURGERY: That type of surgery performed on the brain in order to alleviate pain, to control violent behavior, occasionally to aid in the treatment of mental illness.

PSYCHOTHERAPY: That specific form of treatment of an individual which is a talking therapy, helping the individual come to grips with his internal conflicts and deal effectively with them. There are many forms and types of psychotherapy. Most psychotherapy today is based on early Freudian concepts and is called psychoanalytically oriented psychotherapy, helping the individual to understand his unconscious conflicts. A more recent form of psychotherapy is behavior therapy which does not concern itself with early psychological conflicts or childhood difficulties but is primarily geared toward helping the individual overcome his anxieties which keep him from functioning effectively.

RATIONALIZATION: A defense mechanism which people use to excuse behavior or to help understand or justify it.

REACTION FORMATION: A defense mechanism characterized by acting against one's fears. For example, one may be very much afraid of heights, and as a reaction formation he may learn to become a pilot or a mountain climber.

REACTIVE DEPRESSION: Another name for a neurotic depression but is of a reactive type; i.e. it is not endogenous but reactive to external circumstances and stimuli.

REALITY PRINCIPLE: That principle which deals with reality and refers to the actual surroundings, rather than the solipsistic or internal idiosyncratic concerns of the individual.

RECIDIVISM: The recurrence of aberrant behavior, usually of a criminal type. A person is said to be a recidivist if he repeats certain crimes.

RECURRENT: An illness is said to recur if it returns; a reaction that has subsided also may recur.

REGRESSION: A dynamic mechanism of returning to an earlier stage of one's development, often under the stress of trauma or illness. The regression may be in the service of the ego; i.e. it may help the individual to survive, or it may be a pathological regression.

REMISSION: An illness is said to be in remission if the acute symptoms have subsided and an individual is not actively psychotic or acutely ill. The term remission implies an interval between acute attacks.

RESISTANCE: That emotional defense which keeps people from getting too close to their own internal conflicts. A person is resistant to the uncovering of conflicts which are painful to him.

SADISM: Refers to the desire to hurt others. Enjoyment or pleasure derived from harming others, specifically in sexual relationships.

SCHIZOID: That label used for an individual who is not schizophrenic or psychotic but who is bizarre and unusual in his behavior. He is in touch with reality but he is socially withdrawn, isolated and has poor relationships with others.

SCHIZOPHRENIA: A major mental illness in which the patient, when acutely ill, is not in touch with reality. Schizophrenia may have recurrences and remissions. A person may have a diagnosis of schizophrenia and not be actively psychotic at the time. It is a functional illness of major proportions which is characterized primarily by a thought disorder rather than an affective disorder such as depression or mania. The four types of schizophrenia that are described are *paranoid*, a person who has delusions of reference, either grandiose or persecutory; *hebephrenic*, a silly, regressed individual who is not in touch with reality; *catatonic*, characterized by waxy flexibility, slow or limited movements and silence; *simple*, a type of schizophrenia which does not have any of those hallmarks but is characterized primarily by being out of touch with reality. The *simple* schizophrenic often is found on Skid Row.

SECONDARY GAIN: That emotional gain an individual achieves from certain symptoms. The secondary gain, e.g. in an hysterical paralysis may be the emotional compensation for not assuming various responsibilities or the monetary award he would receive.

SENSORIUM: That part of the individual that takes in the stimuli from the outside. It is usually considered to be a part of the brain rather than the mind.

SEXUAL DEVIATION: Originally, any act that was not peno-vaginal intercourse between a male and a female as the primary mode of sexual expression was considered to be a sexual deviation. The liberalization of sexual conduct has influenced psychiatrists to feel that sexual deviation ought to be limited to those forms of sexual expression which are used exclusively to avoid peno-vaginal intercourse except for consensual homosexual behavior. Homosexuality is considered by some to be an alternation, rather than a deviation of normal sexual expression. Primarily sadomasochism, pedophilia and other harmful behavior to others are considered to be deviations. Some of the deviations are exhibitionism, voyeurism, frottage, pedophilia, rape, bestiality, zoophilia and necrophilia.

SHOCK THERAPY: Electroshock therapy which is used primarily for the treatment of serious depression.

SIGN: That objective change in an individual's physical or emotional health which is aberrant and a sign of illness. A sign as opposed to a symptom, is something the physician observes rather than that which the patient feels and tells the doctor about.

SOCIOPATH: Another name for psychopath or antisocial personality. The name refers to an individual who does not learn from previous experiences, has a defect in his conscience and usually acts out his internal conflicts, often getting into difficulty with the law.

SOMATIZATION: Refers to the physical symptoms found in individuals with emotional conflicts. It is a way of shifting the emotional conflict to the physical systems. Thus a psychosomatic illness such as an ulcer may represent a somatization of the emotional conflict to the stomach.

SUBLIMATION: A defense mechanism by which one handles anxiety by sublimating internal conflicts into socially acceptable means of behaving. For example, an individual who is dealing with hostile, angry, murderous impulses may be very successful as a butcher and may take great pleasure and gratification in cutting up meat and dismembering animals.

SUPEREGO: That conscience which develops through identification with authority figures and tells the individual not to do certain things; it is the "no-no"; it is the control over the id urges.

SUPPRESSION: A conscious putting down, forgetting, of material as opposed to an unconscious forgetting or repression.

SYMPTOM: A subjective feeling on the part of the patient, e.g. pain, discomfort, about which the patient can tell the doctor.

Glossary

SYNDROME: A collection of symptoms that one experiences. It reflects a certain well-recognized illness or set of symptoms.

TOXIC: Refers to poisonous substance or reaction or that which negatively affects an individual; usually a drug or medication.

TRANSFERENCE: That interaction between people which is characterized by an alteration or deviation from reality to some previous relationship the individual has experienced. For example, a person has a transference relationship with his therapist when he considers the therapist to be his father, his mother or brother, because he sees characteristics in the therapist which are similar to those that he experienced with his father, mother or brother, and acts with the therapist accordingly.

TRAUMA: Any negative effect on the body or the mind. A person may be traumatized if he receives a blow anywhere to the body. The trauma will have physical manifestations such as a bruise or cut or bleeding or broken bone, etc. The emotional aspect of trauma is just as real and as measurable and as painful to the individual. Emotional trauma may occur without concomitant physical trauma to the individual. Consider, for example, the trauma a mother experiences when her child is injured.

TRAUMATIC NEUROSIS: A specific psychoneurosis that follows, is related to, and caused by trauma. The cardinal signs of such a traumatic neurosis are social and emotional withdrawal, sexual decrease or abstinence, repetitive dreams of the trauma, trembling, nervousness, anxiety, depressive features, lack of appetite and sleeplessness.

TRUTH SERUM: A misnomer for either sodium amytal or sodium pentothal. There is no such thing as a truth serum or a serum that will make people tell the truth. The barbiturates used in these cases merely lower the threshold for resistance, both conscious and unconscious, and underlying material will be more readily recalled or remembered. However, the psychological effect of calling the material "truth serum" does influence the person receiving it to tell what comes to his mind.

INDEX

A

Aberrant, 5
Abrahamson, 133
Abreaction, 41, 208
Actus Reus, 74
Addict
 addiction, 144
Adolescents
 confidentiality of, 215
 criminal proceedings, 109
Adultery, 171
Adversary, 59, 137
 procedure, 47
Affective, 27
Alcohol
 abuse, 180
 role in violent behavior, 97
Alcoholism, 141, 152
American Academy of Forensic Sciences, 12
American Academy of Psychiatry and the Law, 12, 96
 Bulletin of, 146
American Bar Foundation, 128, 169
American Board of Psychiatry and Neurology, 40
American College of Legal Medicine, 12
American Handbook of Psychiatry, 127
American Law Institute
 Model Penal Code, 30
American Medical Association
 mental disorders, 185
American Psychiatric Association, 31
 State of Ethics, 211
Amnesia, 8, 60
 in criminal matters, 19, 37
 clinical evaluation of, 28
 in trauma, 186
Amphetamines, 142
Annulment, 170
Antisocial personality, 6
Anxiety, 143, 187
 neurosis, 5
Arthur, 67
Aselin, 116
Asthenic personality, 6
Atraumatic, 25

B

Barbiturates, 142
Baughman v. Baughman, 173
Baxstrom, 101
Behaviorists, 95
Birnbaum, M., 178
Blackburn v. U.S., 75
Blackout, 28, 38
Brancale, R., 129
Brandeis, L., 61
Brain damage, 99, 194
Bray v. Bray, 173
Briscoe, C. W., 167

C

Catathymic crisis, 116
Child custody, 22, 159
Civil rights, 165, 177
Combat fatigue, 188
Commitment, 13, 78, 177
Commonwealth v. Hipple, 64
Community Legal Services, 179
Compensation
 as a defense mechanism, 8
 Workmen's, 18
Competency, 14, 151

247

evaluation of, 27
  in criminal matters, 79
Concussion, cerebral, 192
Confession
  statements, 27
  voluntary, 76
Confidentiality, 211
Consciousness
  altered state of, 38
Conversion, 186
Coprophilia, 127
Court order, 32
Criminal behavior, 214
  responsibility, 73
Currens test, 30
Cyclothymic personality, 6

D

Dangerousness, 83, 165
  prediction of, 95
Danto, B., 146
Dawidoff, D. J., 210
Depression
  depressive neurosis, 5
Desensitization, 9
Determinism, 9
Deviations, list of, 127
Diagnosis, 10
Diagnostic impression, 31
Diagnostic and Statistical Manual (DSM-II), 6
Diamond, B., 80
Dilantin, 97
Diplomate in Psychiatry, 40
Domestic relations, 22, 159
  Law, 169
Due process clause, 111
Dynamicists, 96

E

E.E.G. (Electroencephalogram), 190, 194
  abnormal, 99
Ellis, 129
Epilepsy, 97
Episodic dyscontrol, 97

Execution
  stay of, 74
Exhibitionism, 127
Explosive personality, 6

F

Flashback phenomena, 145
Fenichel, 135
Fetishism, 127
Frankfurter, F., 68
Freud, S., 8, 135

G

Gault Decision, 110
Gersen & Victoroff, 66
Glueck, S. & E., 96
Goldstein, A. S., 77
Goldzband, M., 97
Gray & Mohr, 132
Group for Advancement of Psychiatry (GAP), 120, 212
Guttmacher, M., 61, 63, 82
  and Weihofen, 131

H

Habeas corpus, 77, 178
Hadfield Case, 99
Hallucinations, 87, 156
Hashish, 87
Heller, M. S., 96
Heroin, 91, 144
Homosexual
  act, 105
  fantasies, 217
  latent, 39
  panic, 39
  perversion, 127
House, T. S., 59
Hypnosis, 60
Hypochondriac neurosis, 5
Hypothetical question, 56
Hysteria, 186
  hysterical personality, 186
  conversion, 184
  features, 168

I

Imminent danger, 211
Inadequate personality, 6
Inbau, 62
Indignities, 172
Informed consent, 206, 212-219
Insanity defense, 33, 78, 81
    related to domestic relations, 170, 171, 174
Intrapsychic conflicts, 95

J

Juvenile court statute, 109

K

Karpman, 134
Koessler, M., 65
Kozol, H., 97
Kraepelin, 133
Krafft-Ebing, 133

L

L.S.D., 87, 145
Legal Aid Society, 162
Lie detector, 19, 29, 60, 76
Lithium carbonate, 143
Ludwig, A. O., 65

M

M'Naghten test, 39, 81, 99, 120, 170, 222
Macdonald, J. M., 63, 126
Maletsky, B., 97
Malingering, 28, 60, 186
Malpractice, 13, 102, 205
Manic-depressive psychosis, 10
    medication for, 143
Manley v. Manley, 170-171
Marijuana, 16, 144, 215
Matchin v. Matchin, 172
Matricide, 117
Mecir, 116
Mens rea, 74
Mentally disabled, 169

Mentally retarded, 157
Mental status examination, 26, 74, 190
Mind-body dichotomy, 6
Modlin, H. C., 187
Morris, T., 117

N

Narcoanalysis, 62
Narcotics, 142
Necrophilia, 127
National Institute of Mental Health, 13
Negligence, 15
Neurological tests, 190
Neuropsychiatrist, 9
Neuroses, list of, 5
Neurosis
    compensation, 188
    hysterical, 6, 186
    personal injury, 188
    post-traumatic, 187-188
    traumatic, 188
    triggered, 188
Non compos mentis, 158, 173
Noyes, A., 7

O

Obsessive-compulsive
    neurosis, 6, 193
    personality, 6
O'Connell, 117
Organic etiology, 28
Orientation
    in examination, 31

P

Paranoid personality, 6
Parens patria, 109
Parole, 102, 216
Parricide, 98, 116
Passive-aggressive personality, 6
Pathological, 195
Patricide, 117
Pavlovian conditioning, 9
Pedophilia, 127
People v. Esposito, 64
People v. Hector, 134

People v. Jones, 64
People v. Leyra, 76
Perr, I., 207
Personality disorders
 list of, 6
Perversion, 127
Peters, J. J., 99
Phobia
 phobic neurosis, 5
 reaction, 196
Plaintiff, 198
 in tort action, 22
Polygraph (see lie detector)
Post-traumatic neurosis, 193
Pregenital, 135
Presentence investigation, 82, 137
Privilege, 211
Psychedelics, 142
Psychiatry, 5
 American Handbook of, 127
 and insurance, 217
Psychic injury, examination for, 189
Psychoanalysis
 and confidentiality, 211
 concepts, 8
Psychological testing, 19, 27, 120, 221
Psychopathic personality, 129
Psychopath, sexual, 128
Psychophysiological reactions, 187
Psychosis, 5, 152, 185
 chronic, 175
 medication for, 143
Psychotic reaction, acute, 181

R

Rape, 127, 136
Rappeport, J., 12, 96
Recidivistic offenses, 138
Redlich, F. C., 66
Regression, 7
 defense mechanism, 8
Repression, 8, 28, 29
Res ipsa loquitur, 206
Responsibility, criminal, 14, 19, 31, 73
Robitscher, J., 188
Rouse v. Cumsron, 178
Rubin, B., 96

S

Sadomasochism, 127
Schizoid personality, 6
Schizophrenia, 5
 paranoid, 39, 99
Scopolamine, 59
Secondary gain neurosis, 187
Seizures, 99
Sexual offender, 127
Sexual psychopath statutes, 83, 128
Shoplifting, 16
Silving, H., 62
Sociopath, 11, 129
 and disability, 185
Sodium amytal, 19, 29, 38, 59, 76
Sodium pentothal, 59
Sodomy, 127
Stress, 7
Stutte, H., 4
Subpoena of records, 15
Suicide, 15, 207
Szasz, T., 61

T

Tappan, 131
Tenney, 138
Testamentary capacity, 152
Testimony, psychiatric, 35, 47, 80
Therapy
 behavior, 9
 chemo, 9
 electroshock, 9, 206
 group and confidentiality, 213
Torts, 22
Tranquilizers, 142
Transvestitism, 127
Trauma, 184
Treatment
 right to, 178
Truth serum, *see* Sodium amytal

U

Unconsciousness, 189
Ungerleider, T., 145

V

Vereeckin, J. L., 116
Violence, 95
Visitation, 22, 159
Voyeurism, 127

W

Wahl, C. W., 218
Watson, A., 8
Weihofen, H., 131
Wertham, F., 116

Whitaker, C. A., 166
Withdrawal
　from drugs, 144
　social, 187

X

XYY chromosomes, 97

Z

Zoophilia, 127